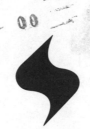

Stedman's

ENT
WORDS

SANS
TACHE

Williams & Wilkins

BALTIMORE • PHILADELPHIA • HONG KONG
LONDON • MUNICH • SYDNEY • TOKYO

A WAVERLY COMPANY

Series Editor: Elizabeth Randolph
Editor: Jocelyn Jenik-Black
Production Coordinators: Barbara Felton, Kim Nawrozki
Cover Design: Carla Frank

Copyright © 1993
Williams & Wilkins
428 East Preston Street
Baltimore, Maryland 21202, USA

Printed in the United States of America

Library of Congress Cataloging-in-Publication Data
Stedman's ENT words.
    p. cm.
    Developed from Stedman's medical dictionary, 25th ed. and supplemented by terminology found in the current medical literature.
    Includes bibliographical references.
    ISBN 0-683-07963-8
    1. Otolaryngology—Terminology.   I. Stedman, Thomas Lathrop, 1853–1938.   Medical dictionary.   II. Title: ENT words.
    [DNLM: 1. Otolarynology—terminology.   WV 13 S8117 1993]
RF24.S74   1993
617.5'1'0014—dc20
DNLM/DLC
for Library of Congress   93-17042
                                                                          CIP

                                                                          97
                                                        6   7   8   9   10

Contents

ACKNOWLEDGMENTS v

EXPLANATORY NOTES vii

A-Z ENT WORD LIST........................... 1

APPENDICES...................................... A1

Acknowledgments

An important part of our editorial process is the involvement of medical transcriptionists—as advisors, reviewers and/or editors. Jocelyn Jenik-Black did an excellent job of editing and proofing the manuscript. Special thanks go to Barbara Eades, Terri Wakefield, CMT and Averill Ring, CMT, who perused texts, journals, and manufacturer's information to compile an up-to-date base of ENT terms.

Also, as with all our Stedman's word references, we have benefited from the suggestions and expertise of our many contacts in the medical transcriptionist community. Thanks to all our advisory board participants, reviewers and editors, AAMT meeting attendees, and others who have written in with requests and comments—keep talking, and we'll keep listening.

Explanatory Notes

Stedman's ENT Words offers an authoritative assurance of quality and exactness to the wordsmiths of the health care professions— medical transcriptionists, medical editors and copy editors, medical records personnel, and the many other users and producers of medical documentation. **Stedman's ENT Words** can be used to validate both the spelling and accuracy of terminology in otorhinolaryngology. This compilation of over 15,000 entries, fully cross-indexed for quick access, was built from a base vocabulary of 10,000 medical words, phrases, abbreviations and acronyms. The extensive A-Z list was developed from the database of **Stedman's Medical Dictionary, 25ed**. and supplemented by terminology found in the current medical literature.

Medical transcription is an art as well as a science. Both are needed to correctly interpret a physician's dictation, whose language is a product of education, training, and experience. This variety in medical language means that there are several acceptable ways to express certain terms, including jargon. **Stedman's ENT Words** provides variant spellings and phrasings for many terms. This, in addition to complete cross-indexing, makes **Stedman's ENT Words** a valuable resource for determining the validity of ENT terms as they are encountered.

Stedman's ENT Words includes up-to-date terminology of otorhinolaryngology (ENT); head and neck surgery; maxillofacial and reconstructive surgery; bronchoesophagology; and communicative disorders. The user will find listed thousands of diseases and syndromes, diagnostic and surgical procedures, and equipment, instrument and device names. Abbreviations and medications pertaining to ENT are also included.

Alphabetical Organization

Alphabetization of entries is letter by letter as spelled, ignoring punctuation, spaces, prefixed numbers, Greek letters, or other characters. For example:

> **acid-fast staining methods**
> **acid formaldehyde hematin**
> α_1**-acid glycoprotein**
> **acid hematin**

In subentries, the abbreviated singular form or the spelled-out plural form of the noun main entry word is ignored in alphabetization.

Format and Style

All main entries are in **boldface** to speed up location of a sought-after entry, to enhance distinction between main entries and sub-entries, and to relieve the textual density of the pages.

Irregular plurals and variant spellings are shown on the same line as the singular or preferred form of the word. For example:

> **fossa,** gen. and pl. **fossae**
> **sialadenitis, sialoadenitis.**

Possessive forms that occur in the medical literature are retained in this reference. It should be noted, however, that equipment and instrument names usually appear in the non-possessive. To form the non-possessives advocated by the American Association for Medical Transcription and other groups, simply drop the apostrophe or apostrophe "s" from the end of the word.

Cross-indexing

The word list is in an index-like main entry-subentry format that contains two combined alphabetical listings:

(1) A noun main entry-subentry organization typical of the A-Z section of medical dictionaries like **Stedman's**:

agnosia	**cyst**
acoustic a.	arachnoid c.
auditory a.	branchial c.
auditory-verbal a.	bronchogenic c.
finger a.	dentigerous c.
tactile a.	globulomaxillary c.

(2) An adjective main entry-subentry organization, which lists words and phrases as you hear them. The main entries are the adjectives or modifiers descriptors in a multi-word term. The subentries are the nouns around which the terms are constructed and to which the adjectives or descriptors pertain:

acetone	**endometrial**
a. body	e. curettage
a. compound	e. cyst
a. fixative	e. hyperplasia
a. text	e. polyp

This format provides the user with more than one way to locate and identify a multi-word term. For example:

drill	**Osteon**
Osteon air d.	O. air drill

amino acid	**glucogenic**
glucogenic a. a.	g. amino acid
ketogenic a. a.	
modified a. a.	

It also allows the user to see together all terms that contain a particular descriptor as well as all types, kinds, or variations of a noun entity. For example:

otitis
aviation o.
o. desquamativa
o. diphtheritica
o. externa hemorrhagica
o. media
reflux o. media
serous o.

Wherever possible, abbreviations are separately defined and cross-referenced. For example:

BPPV
benign paroxysmal positional vertigo
benign
b. paroxysmal positional vertigo (BPPV)
vertigo
benign paroxysmal positional v. (BPPV)

References

Ballenger, Diseases of the nose, throat, ear, head and neck, 14ed. Malvern: Lea & Febiger, 1991.

Georgiade, Textbook of plastic, maxillofacial, and reconstructive surgery, 2ed. Baltimore: Williams & Wilkins; 1992.

Grannick, Management of salivary gland lesions. Baltimore: Williams & Wilkins; 1992.

The hearing journal. Baltimore: Williams & Wilkins; 1992–93.

Mehta, Atlas of endoscopic sinonasal surgery. Malvern: Lea & Febiger; 1992.

Nicolosi, Terminology of communicative disorders, 4ed. Baltimore: Williams & Wilkins; 1990.

Otolaryngology-head and neck surgery. St. Louis: Mosby-Yearbook; 1992–3.

Silverstein, Surgical techniques of the temporal bone and skull base. Malvern: Lea & Febiger; 1992.

Swartz, Head and neck microsurgery. Baltimore: Williams & Wilkins; 1992.

Your Medical Word Resource Publisher

We strive to provide you with the most up-to-date and accurate word references available. Your use of this word book will prompt new editions, which will be published as often as justified by updates and revisions. We welcome your suggestions for improvements, changes, corrections, and additions—whatever will make this **Stedman's** product more useful to you. Please use the postpaid card at the back of this book and send your recommendations to the Reference Division at Williams & Wilkins.

A
　　ampere
AAMD
　　American Association On
　　　Mental Deficiency
ABA
　　Apraxia Battery for Adults
abdomen
abdominal
　　a. adipose tissue
abducent
　　a. nerve
abduction
abductor paralysis
aberrant
ability
　　central auditory a.'s
　　Flowers-Costello Test of
　　　Central Auditory A.'s
　　Illinois Test of
　　　Psycholinguistic A.'s
　　　(ITPA)
　　McCarthy Scales of
　　　Children's A.'s
　　Porch Index of
　　　Communicative A.'s
　　　(PICA)
　　a. test
ABL520 blood gas measurement
　system
ablative procedure
ABLB
　　Alternate Binaural Loudness
　　　Balance
abnormal
abnormality
　　clotting a.
ABR
　　auditory brainstem response
abrupt topic shift
abscess
　　apical a.
　　brain a.
　　cerebellar a.
　　epidural a.
　　extradural a.
　　laryngeal a.
　　lung a.
　　masseter a.
　　nasal septal a.

　　nasopharyngeal a.
　　orbital a.
　　parapharyngeal space a.
　　parotid gland a.
　　perisinus a.
　　peritonsillar a.
　　prevertebral space a.
　　retropharyngeal a.
　　stellate a.
　　subdural a.
　　subperiosteal a.
　　temporal fossa a.
　　temporal lobe a.
absent epiglottis
absolute
　　a. construction
　　a. quantity
　　a. threshold
absorption
abstraction
　　a. ladder
abulia
abuse
　　vocal a.
abusive vocal behavior
abutting consonant
AC
　　air conduction
　　alternating current
acalculia
Acanthamoeba
acatamathesia
acataphasia
accelerated speech
acceleration
　　interverbal a.
　　intraverbal a.
accelerometer
accent
　　foreign a.
accessory
　　a. maxillary ostium
　　a. ostium
　　a. sinus
accident
　　cerebrovascular a. (CVA)
accommodation
accusative case
ACCUSAT pulse oximeter
ACCUTORR bedside monitor

ACE
    angiotensin-converting enzyme
acetazolamide
acetonide
    triamcinolone a.
acetylcholine
    a. receptor
acetylsalicylic acid
achalasia
achievement
    a. age
    a. quotient (AQ)
achlorhydric anemia
acid
    acetylsalicylic a.
    boric a.
    a. caustic
    cis-retinoic a.
    nicotinic a.
    retinoic a.
acid-hematoxylin
    phosphotungstic a.-h.
    (PTAH)
acidosis
acid-Schiff
    periodic a.-S. (PAS)
acinar cell
acinic
    a. cell carcinoma
    a. cell tumor
acinous cell carcinoma
acinus
aclarubicin
ACLC
    Assessment of Children's
    Language Comprehension
acouesthesia
acoupedic method
acoupedics
acoustic
    a. agnosia
    a. analysis
    a. contralateral reflex
    a. energy
    a. feedback
    a. gain
    a. gain control
    a. immittance measurement
    a. impedance
    a. impedance probe
    a. ipsilateral reflex
    a. macula
    a. meatus

    a. method
    a. nerve
    a. neurilemoma
    a. neurinoma
    a. neuroma
    a. notch
    a. phonetics
    a. pressure
    a. reflex
    a. reflex amplitude
    a. reflex decay
    a. reflex latency
    a. reflex pattern
    a. reflex threshold
    a. schwannoma
    a. spectrum
    a. stapedial reflex
    a. stria
acoustica
    hyperesthesia a.
acoustic-amnestic aphasia
acousticopalpebral reflex
acquired
    a. aphasia
    a. cholesteatoma
    a. immunodeficiency
    syndrome (AIDS)
acral lentiginous melanoma
acrolect
acromegaly
act
    biological a.
    sensorimotor a.
    speech a.
actin
actinic keratosis
Actinomyces
    A. bovis
    A. israelii
    A. naeslundii
actinomycosis
action-locative
action-object
action potential
activation
active
    a. bilingualism
    a. filter
    a. voice
acuity
    auditory a.
    olfactory a.

a. test
visual a.
Acuspot
710 A.
Sharplan Laser 710 A.
acusticus
porus a.
acute
a. diffuse external otitis
a. follicular adenoiditis
a. frontal sinusitis
a. laryngitis
a. localized external otitis
a. maxillary sinusitis
a. necrotizing ulcerative
gingivitis (ANUG)
a. otitis media (AOM)
a. phoneme
a. respiratory disease
a. suppurative parotitis
a. supraglottic laryngitis
acyclovir
adamantinoma
Adam's apple
adaptation
auditory a.
a. effect
a. test
Adaptic gauze
adaptive
a. behavior
a. immunity
ADCC
antibody-dependent cellular
cytotoxicity
ADD
attention deficit disorder
Addison's disease
adduction
adductor
a. longus muscle

a. magnus muscle
a. paralysis
a. spasmodic dysphonia
adenitis
tuberculous a.
adenocarcinoma
bronchial a.
gastrointestinal a.
mucinous cell a.
papillary a.
polymorphous low-grade a.
(PLGA)
prostatic a.
adenoid
a. cystic carcinoma
a. cystic tumor
a. facies
lateral trim of the a.
a. squamous carcinoma
adenoidal pad
adenoidectomy
lateral a.
tonsillectomy and a. (T&A)
adenoiditis
acute follicular a.
follicular a.
hyperplastic a.
hypertrophic a.
recurrent bacterial a.
adenolymphoma
adenolymphomatosum
adenoma
basaloid monomorphic a.
(BMA)
bronchial a.
carcinoma expleomorphic a.
duodenal a.
monomorphic a.
oxyphilic a.
parathyroid a.
pleomorphic a.

NOTES

adenoma *(continued)*
  sebaceous a.
  thyroid a.
  tracheal a.
adenomatous polyp
adenopapillary carcinoma
adenosine triphosphate (ATP)
adenotonsillar
adenotonsillectomy
adenovirus
ADHD
  attention deficit hyperactivity
    disorder
adherence
  immune a.
adhesive
  a. otitis media
  silicone a.
adiadochokinesis
adipose tissue
adjuvant chemotherapy
adolescent
  Fullerton Language Test
    for A.'s
  A. Language Screening Test
  a. voice
β-adrenergic
α-adrenergic
adrenocorticotropic hormone
Adriamycin
Adson forceps
adult
  Apraxia Battery for A.'s
    (ABA)
  Slosson Intelligence Test for
    Children and A.'s
advancement flap
adventitious
  a. deafness
AED
  aerodynamic equivalent
    diameter
AERA
  average evoked response
    audiometry
aeration
aerobic bacteria
aerodigestive
  a. tract
  a. tumor
aerodynamic
  a. analysis

  a. equivalent diameter
    (AED)
aerodynamics
aerophagia
aerotitis media
aeruginosa
  Pseudomonas a.
affective function
afferent
  a. feedback
  a. motor aphasia
  a. nerve
affricate
affrication
affricative
after-glide
age
  achievement a.
  basal a.
  chronological a. (CA)
  developmental a.
  educational a. (EA)
  mental a. (MA)
agenesis
  tracheal a.
agenitive
agent
  alkylating a.
  anesthetic a.
  antineoplastic a.
  antipseudomonal a.
  hypotensive a.
  immunosuppressive a.
  paralytic a.
  vasoconstrictive a.
agent-action
agent-object
agger nasi cell
agitolalia
aglossia
agnathia
agnosia
  acoustic a.
  auditory a.
  auditory verbal a.
  finger a.
  tactile a.
  visual a.
  visual-verbal a.
agonist
agrammalogia, agrammatologia
agrammatica
agrammatism

agrammatologia (*var. of*
  agrammalogia)
agraphia
  pure a.
AHH
  arylhydrocarbon hydroxylase
aid
  air-conduction hearing a.
  binaural hearing a.
  body hearing a.
  bone-conduction hearing a.
  canal hearing a.
  compression hearing a.
  digital hearing a.
  hearing a.
  interoral speech a.
  in-the-ear hearing a.
  linear hearing a.
  monaural hearing a.
  pseudobinaural hearing a.
  Servox electronic speech a.
  Servox Inton speech a.
  Trilogy I hearing a.
  vibrotactile hearing a.
  Y-cord hearing a.
aided augmentative communication
AIDS
  acquired immunodeficiency
    syndrome
AIDS-related complex (ARC)
air
  a. cell
  complemental a.
  a. conduction (AC)
  a. embolism
  a. embolus
  a. flow
  a. injection
  ionized a.
  a. pollutant
  reserve a.

residual a.
a. space
supplemental a.
tidal a.
a. wastage
air-blade sound
air-bone gap
air-conduction
  a.-c. hearing aid
  a.-c. receiver
air-iodinated contrast
airstream
  nasal a.
airway
  a. management
  nasal a.
  a. obstruction
  upper a.
AJCC
  American Joint Committee for
  Cancer
Akros mattress
ala, pl. **alae**
  nasal a.
  a. nasi
alalia
alar
  a. base
  a. base reduction
  a. cartilage
  a. facial groove
  a. flutter
  a. muscle
  a. reconstruction
  a. wedge excision
alaryngeal
  a. speech
albicans
  Candida a.
Albrecht syndrome
albumin

NOTES

5

alcohol
    isopropyl a.
ALD
    Appraisal of Language
    Disturbance
aldosterone
alexia
    auditory a.
    pure a.
    visual a.
alkali caustic
alkaline phosphatase
alkylating agent
All Access laser system
Allen's test
Allen traction system
Allergen
allergen
Allergen Ear Drops
allergic sialadenitis
allergy
alligator forceps
alliteration
allomorph
allophone
alloplastic transplant
allusion
alogia
alpha
    a. rhythm
    a. wave
alphabet
    initial teaching a.
    International Phonetic A.
    (IPA)
    International Standard
      Manual A.
    manual a.
    phonetic a.
ALPS
    Aphasia Language Performance
    Scale
ALS
    amyotrophic lateral sclerosis
alternate
    A. Binaural Loudness
      Balance (ABLB)
    a. forms reliability
      coefficient
    A. Monaural Loudness
      Balance (AMLB)
    a. motion rate (AMR)

alternating
    a. current (AC)
    a. pulse
alternative communication
Alton Deal pressure infusor
alveolar
    a. area
    a. artery
    a. carcinoma
    a. hyperventilation
    a. hypoventilation
    a. nerve
    a. process
    a. ridge
Alzheimer's disease
AM
    amplitude modulation
amalgam
    dental a.
ambidextrous
ambient noise
ambiguous, ambiguus
    nucleus a.
    a. word
ambilaterality
ambisyllabic
ambivalence
ambiversion
amebic infection
ameloblastoma
amentia
Americaine Otic ear drops
American
    A. Association On Mental
      Deficiency (AAMD)
    A. Indian Sign Language
      (AMERIND)
    A. Joint Committee for
      Cancer (AJCC)
    A. Medical Source
      laparoscopic equipment
    A. National Standards
      Institute (ANSI)
    A. Sign Language (Ameslan,
      ASL)
    A. Speech-Language-Hearing
      Association (ASHA)
    A. Standards Association
      (ASA)
AMERIND
    American Indian Sign Language
Ameslan
    American Sign Language

amimia
aminoglycoside
AMLB
  Alternate Monaural Loudness
  Balance
Ammons Full Range Picture
  Vocabulary Test
amnesia
  localized a.
  posttraumatic a. (PTA)
  retroactive a.
amnesic, amnestic
  a. aphasia
ampere (A)
amphotericin B
ampicillin
  a. sodium
amplification
  compression a.
amplifier
amplify
amplitude
  acoustic reflex a.
  a. distortion
  effective a.
  maximum a.
  a. modulation (AM)
  a. shimmer
  zero a.
ampulla
  membranaceous a.
  osseous a.
ampullaris
  crista a.
ampullary
  a. crest
  a. nerve
AMR
  alternate motion rate
amusia

amylacea
  corpora a.
amylase
α-amylase ptyalin
amyloidosis
amyotrophic lateral sclerosis (ALS)
anacusis, anacousis, anakusis
anaerobic bacteria
analog
  testosterone a.
analogy
analysis, pl. analyses
  acoustic a.
  aerodynamic a.
  auditory a.
  distinctive feature a.
  Fourier a.
  grammatical a.
  kinesthetic a.
  kinetic a.
  perceptual a.
  phonemic a.
  phonetic a.
  phonological a.
  phonological process a.
  segmental a.
  sound a.
  substitution a.
  suprasegmental a.
  task a.
  traditional a.
analytic method
analyzer
  noise a.
  octave band a.
anaphoric
  a. pronoun
anaphylactic shock
anaptyxis, pl. anaptyxes
anarthria

NOTES

anastomosis
   end-to-side a.
   Galen's a.
   lymphaticovenous a.
   microvascular a.
   nerve a.
   Roux-en-Y a.
Andrews spinal surgery table
androsterone sulfate
Andy Gump deformity
anechoic chamber
anemia
   achlorhydric a.
anemometer
   warm-wire a.
anesthesia
   cocaine a.
   general a.
   intracavitary a.
   laryngeal a.
   local a.
   regional a.
   topical a.
anesthetic
   a. agent
   local a.
   Silverstein tetracaine base
     powder a.
aneurysm
   aortic a.
   basilar artery a.
   carotid a.
   posterior fossa artery a.
angina
   Ludwig's a.
   pseudomembranous a.
   Vincent's a.
angiofibroma
   juvenile nasopharyngeal a.
   nasopharyngeal a.
angiography
   magnetic resonance a.
   (MRA)
angioleiomyoma
   laryngeal a.
angioma
angiomatous neoplastic tissue
angioneurotic edema
angiosarcoma
angiotensin-converting enzyme
   (ACE)
angle
   auriculomastoid a.

   cerebellopontine a. (CPA)
   cerebropalatine a.
   cricothyroid a.
   sinodural a.
   visor a.
angled telescope
Angle's classification
angular
   a. artery
   a. facial vein
   a. gyrus
   a. vein
   a. vestibular nucleus
angulated cell
animate
ankyloglossia
ankylosing spondylitis
ankylosis
   bony a.
   cricoarytenoid a.
annular ligament
annulus
   bony a.
   tympanic a.
   a. tympanicus
anode
anomalous
anomaly
   craniofacial a.
   laryngeal a.
anomia
anomic
   a. aphasia
anosmia
anosognosia
anoxia
   cerebral a.
ansa
   a. galeni
   a. hypoglossi
   a. hypoglossus muscle
anserinus
   pes a.
ANSI
   American National Standards
   Institute
antagonist
   narcotic a.
antegrade approach
anterior
   a. clinoid process
   a. commissure
   a. cricoid split

a. ethmoid
a. ethmoidal air cell
a. ethmoidal artery
a. ethmoidal foramen
a. ethmoid artery
a. ethmoidectomy
a. ethmoid nerve
a. ethmoid ostium
a. facial vein
a. helical rim free flap
a. mallear fold
a. mallear ligament
a. naris
a. nasal spine
a. nasal valve
a. partial laryngectomy
a. rectus capitis
rhinitis sicca a.
a. suspensory ligament
a. tympanic artery
a. vertical canal
anterosuperior quadrant
anthelix
anthrax
anthropological linguistics
anthropometric measurement
antibiotic
　intravenous a.
　IV a.
　oral a.
antibody
　antiductal a.
　antinuclear a.
　anti-Ro a.'s
　collagen a.
　monoclonal a.
　radiolabeled a.
　salivary gland a.
　smooth muscle a.
　thyroglobulin a.

antibody-dependent cellular cytotoxicity (ADCC)
anticholinergic
anticholinesterase
anticipatory
　a. coarticulation
　a. reaction
　a. and struggle behavior theories
anticoagulant
anticonvulsive drug
anticus
　isthmus tympani a.
antiductal antibody
anti-expectancy
antigen
　HLA a.
　a. receptor
　Ro intracellular a.
　tumor-specific a.
antigen-presenting cell
antihelix
antihistamine
antihormonal therapy
anti-idiotype
antimesenteric
antimetabolite
antimicrobial
antimitotic
antineoplastic agent
antinuclear antibody
antipseudomonal agent
antiresonance
antiretroviral therapy
anti-Ro antibodies
antitragohelicina
　fissura a.
antitragus
antral
　a. cell

NOTES

antral *(continued)*
    a. irrigation
    a. lavage
antrochoanal polyp
antrostomy
    inferior meatal a.
    inferior meatus a.
    middle meatal a.
    nasal a.
antrum
    bipartite a.
    a. of Highmore
    mastoid a.
    maxillary a.
ANUG
    acute necrotizing ulcerative
    gingivitis
anvil
anxiety
AOM
    acute otitis media
aorta
aortic
    a. aneurysm
    a. body
8AP
    eighth nerve action potential
apathy
aperiodic
    a. wave
aperiodicity
aperture
    piriform a.
apex, pl. **apices**
    a. nasi
    orbital a.
Apgar Score
aphasia
    acoustic-amnestic a.
    acquired a.
    afferent motor a.
    amnesic a.
    anomic a.
    auditory a.
    Bedside Evaluation and
      Screening Test of A.
    Broca's a.
    central a.
    childhood a.
    A. Clinical Battery I
    conduction a.
    developmental a.
    dynamic a.

efferent motor a.
executive a.
expressive a.
expressive-receptive a.
fluent a.
global a.
infantile a.
International Test for A.
isolation a.
jargon a.
kinesthetic motor a.
kinetic motor a.
Language Modalities Test
  for A.
A. Language Performance
  Scale (ALPS)
Minnesota Test for
  Differential Diagnosis
  of A.
motor a.
nominal a.
nonfluent a.
pragmatic a.
receptive a.
semantic a.
sensory a.
simple a.
speech reading a.
subcortical motor a.
syntactic a.
Token Test for Receptive
  Disturbances in A.
transcortical sensory a.
verbal a.
Wernicke's a.
aphasic
    a. phonological impairment
aphasiologist
aphasiology
aphemia
    pure a.
aphonia
    conversion a.
    functional a.
    hysterical a.
    intermittent a.
    psychogenic a.
    syllabic a.
aphonic
    a. episode
aphrasia
    pure a.

aphthae
    periadenitis a.
apical
    a. abscess
    a. cell
apicalization
apicectomy
    petrous a.
apices (*pl. of* apex)
aplasia
    cochlear a.
apnea
    peripheral a.
    sleep a.
aponeurosis, pl. aponeuroses
apoplexy
apparatus
    vestibular a.
appendix of laryngeal ventricle
apperception
apple
    Adam's a.
application
    topical a.
applied
    a. linguistics
    a. phonetics
appositive
Appraisal of Language Disturbance (ALD)
approach
    antegrade a.
    cochleovestibular a.
    extralaryngeal a.
    infralabyrinthine a.
    infratemporal fossa a.
    middle fossa a.
    otomicrosurgical
      transtemporal a.
    retrograde a.
    retrolabyrinthine a.

    retrosigmoid a.
    suboccipital a.
    supratentorial a.
    transcanine a.
    transcervical a.
    transcochlear a.
    translabyrinthine a.
    transmastoid a.
    transmeatal a.
    transseptal a.
    yawn-sigh a.
approach-avoidance
    a.-a. theory
approximation
    successive a.
    vocal fold a.
    word a.
APR
    auropalpebral reflex
apraxia
    A. Battery for Adults (ABA)
    constructional a.
    oral a.
    speech a.
    verbal a.
apraxic
apron flap
aprosody
apsithyria
aptitude
    Hiskey-Nebraska Test of Learning A.
    a. test
AQ
    achievement quotient
aqueduct
    cerebral a.
    cochlear a.
    vestibular a.
aqueous humor

NOTES

11

arabinosyl
cytosine a.
Ara-C
arachidic bronchitis
arachidonic acid pathy
arachnoid
a. cyst
a. space
ARC
AIDS-related complex
arc
reflex a.
sensorimotor a.
arcade
mesenteric a.
arch
branchial a.
dental a.
glossopalatine a.
hyoid branchial a.
mandibular a.
maxillary a.
pharyngopalatine a.
zygomatic a.
architecture
neural a.
arcuata
eminentia a.
arcuate
a. eminence
a. fasciculus
area
alveolar a.
articulation a.
auditory a.
bilabial a.
Broca's a.
glottal a.
labiodental a.
lingua-alveolar a.
linguodental a.
Little's a.
motor a.
palatal a.
petroclival a.
postauricular a.
prelacrimal a.
somesthetic a.
subglottic a.
velar a.
visual a.
Warthin's a.
Wernicke's a.

areolar tissue
argon
a. laser
a. tuneable dye laser
Argyle
A. anti-reflux valve
A. silicone Salem sump
Army-Navy retractor
Arnold-Bruening syringe
Arnold-Chiari malformation
Arnold's nerve
array
electrode a.
arresting consonant
arrhizus
Rhizopus a.
arrow blade
ARROWgard central venous
catheter
arsenic
arterialized flap
arterial plexus
arteriography
arteriovenous malformation (AVM)
arteritis
giant cell a.
temporal a.
artery
alveolar a.
angular a.
anterior ethmoid a.
anterior ethmoidal a.
anterior tympanic a.
ascending palatine a.
ascending pharyngeal a.
auditory a.
auricular a.
auriculotemporal a.
axillary a.
basilar a.
caroticotympanic a.
carotid a.
circumflex iliac a.
circumflex scapular a.
cochlear a.
common carotid a.
cricothyroid a.
cubital a.
descending palatine a.
dorsal lingual a.
a. of Drummond
epigastric a.
ethmoidal a.

external carotid a.
facial a.
first dorsal metatarsal a.
  (FDMA)
gastroepiploic a.
greater palatine a.
inferior laryngeal a.
inferior thyroid a.
inferior tympanic a.
infrahyoid a.
infraorbital a.
innominate a.
intercostal a.
internal auditory a.
internal carotid a.
internal maxillary a.
laryngeal a.
lesser palatine a.
lingual a.
mammary a.
maxillary a.
medullary a.
meningeal a.
nasal a.
nasal accessory a.
occipital a.
palatine a.
petrosal a.
pharyngeal a.
postauricular a.
posterior auricular a.
posterior ethmoid a.
posterior inferior
  cerebellar a. (PICA)
posterior palatine a.
posterior septal a.
posterior superior
  alveolar a.
posterior tympanic a.
posterolateral nasal a.
profunda femoris a.

radial a.
retroauricular a.
septal a.
sphenopalatine a.
spiral a.
stapedial a.
stylomandibular a.
stylomastoid a.
subscapular a.
superficial petrosal a.
superficial temporal a.
superior alveolar a.
superior laryngeal a.
superior pharyngeal a.
superior thyroid a.
superior tympanic a.
supratrochlear a.
temporal a.
thoracoacromial a.
thoracodorsal a.
thyroid a.
thyroid ima a.
tonsillar a.
transverse cervical a.
transverse facial a.
trigeminal a.
tympanic a.
vertebral a.
vestibulocochlear a.
vidian a.
arthritis
  rheumatoid a.
arthrodesis
  cricoarytenoid a.
arthrogram
**Arthur Adaptation of the Leiter
  International Performance Scale**
articulate
articulation
  a. area

NOTES

articulation *(continued)*
    Assessment Link Between Phonology and A.
    Bryngelson-Glaspey Test of A.
    a. curve
    Deep Test of A.
    deviant a.
    a. disorder
    a. error
    Goldman-Fristoe Test of A.
    a. index
    place of a.
    point of a.
    Predictive Screening Test of A.
    a. programming
    Screening Deep Test of A.
    secondary a.
    Templin-Darley Tests of A.
    a. test
articulation-gain function
articulation-resonance
articulator
articulatory
    a. basis
    a. phonetics
artifact
    background a.
    trigeminal nerve a.
artificial
    a. ear
    a. larynx
    a. mastoid
    a. method
    a. sound generator
    a. tears
aryepiglottic
    a. fold
    a. muscle
arylhydrocarbon hydroxylase (AHH)
arytenoid
    a. cartilage
    a. muscle
    a. perichondritis
arytenoidectomy
ASA
    American Standards Association
asapholalia
ascending
    a. palatine artery
    a. pharyngeal artery

    a. pitch break
    a. process
    a. ramus
    a. ramus of the mandible
    a. technique
asemasia
asemia
aseptic necrosis
ASHA
    American Speech-Language-Hearing Association
ASL
    American Sign Language
aspect
    inferomedial a.
    linguistic a.
    speech a.
aspergillosis
Aspergillus
    A. flavus
    A. fumigatus
    A. niger
aspirate
aspiration
    a. biopsy cytology
    fine-needle a.
    needle a.
    per mucosal needle a.
    a. tube
aspirator
    ULTRA ultrasonic a.
aspirin
assembly
    malleus-footplate a.
    malleus-stapes a.
assessment
    A. of Children's Language Comprehension (ACLC)
    Compton-Hutton Phonological A.
    A. of Intelligibility of Dysarthric Speech
    Interpersonal Language Skills and A. (ILSA)
    A. Link Between Phonology and Articulation
    Performance A. of Syntax Elicited and Spontaneous (PASES)
    A. of Phonological Processes
    System of Multicultural A. (SOMA)

System of Multicultural
Pluralistic A. (SOMPA)
ASSESS peak flow meter
assimilated nasality
assimilation
double a.
labial a.
progressive a.
progressive vowel a.
reciprocal a.
regressive a.
velar a.
association
American Speech-Language-
Hearing A. (ASHA)
American Standards A.
(ASA)
auditory-vocal a.
sound-symbol a.
word a.
assonance
astereognosis
asteroid body
asthenopia
asthma
Millar's a.
astomia
asymmetry
facial a.
asynergia
asynergic
asynergy
ataxia
Friedreich's a.
ataxic
a. dysarthria
atelectasis
atelectatic otitis
athetosis
athetotic

atonia
atopic dermatitis
ATP
adenosine triphosphate
atresia
aural a.
choanal a.
laryngeal a.
oral a.
a. plate
tracheal a.
atrophic rhinitis
atrophy
hemifacial a.
Romberg hemifacial a.
atropine
atropinoid
attachment
Closed Chain Exercise A.
Tasserit shoulder a.
attack
glottal a.
hard glottal a.
transient ischemic a. (TIA)
vocal a.
attention
auditory a.
a. deficit disorder (ADD)
a. deficit hyperactivity
disorder (ADHD)
Flowers Test of Auditory
Selective A.
a. span
attenuation
interaural a.
attenuator
attic cholesteatoma
attribute-entity
atypia
epithelial a.

NOTES

atypical
    a. cleft
    a. mycobacterium
audibility threshold
audible
    a. range
auding
audiogram
    a. configuration
audiologic
    a. habilitation
audiological evaluation
audiologist
audiology
    clinical a.
    diagnostic a.
    educational a.
    experimental a.
    geriatric a.
    pediatric a.
    rehabilitative a.
audiometer
    automatic a.
    Bekesy a.
    group a.
    GSI 16 a.
    limited range a.
    limited range speech a.
    pure-tone a.
    Rudmose a.
    speech a.
    wide range a.
audiometric
    a. test
    a. zero
audiometry
    auditory brainstem
      response a.
    automatic a.
    average evoked response a.
      (AERA)
    behavioral observation a.
      (BOA)
    Bekesy a.
    brainstem-evoked
      response a. (BSER)
    brief tone a. (BTA)
    cardiac-evoked response a.
      (CERA)
    conditioned orientation
      reflex a. (COR)
    delayed feedback a. (DFA)
    diagnostic a.

    electric response a. (ERA)
    electrodermal a. (EDA)
    electrodermal response
      test a. (EDRA)
    electroencephalic a. (EEA)
    electroencephalic response a.
      (ERA)
    evoked response a. (ERA)
    galvanic skin response a.
      (GSRA)
    high frequency a.
    identification a.
    impedance a.
    industrial a.
    live voice a.
    monitored live voice a.
    monitoring a.
    play a.
    psychogalvanic skin
      response a. (PGSRA)
    pure-tone a.
    reduced screening a.
    screening a.
    speech a.
    tangible reinforcement of
      operant conditioned a.
      (TROCA)
    threshold a.
    Visual Reinforcement A.
audito-oculogyric reflex
auditory
    a. acuity
    a. adaptation
    a. agnosia
    a. alexia
    a. analysis
    A. Analysis Test
    a. aphasia
    a. area
    a. artery
    a. attention
    a. blending
    a. brain mapping
    a. brainstem response
      (ABR)
    a. brainstem response
      audiometry
    a. brainstem response test
    a. canal
    a. closure
    a. cortex
    a. cue
    a. differentiation

a. discrimination
A. Discrimination Test
a. disorder
a. fatigue
a. feedback
a. figure-ground
a. figure-ground
  discrimination
a. flutter
a. flutter fusion
a. function
a. imperception
a. localization
a. memory
a. memory span
a. method
a. modality
a. nerve
a. oculogyric response
a. ossicle
a. pathway
a. pattern
a. perception
a. phonetics
A. Pointing Test
a. process
a. processing disorder
a. reflex
a. selective listening
a. sequencing
a. skill
a. synthesis
a. training
a. training units
a. tube
a. vein
a. verbal agnosia
auditory-evoked
  a.-e. potentials
  a.-e. response

auditory-vocal
  a.-v. association
  a.-v. automaticity
augmentative
  a. communication
  a. communication system
aura
aural
  a. atresia
  a. rehabilitation
Aureomycin ointment
aureus
  Staphylococcus a.
auricle
  supernumerary a.
auricular
  a. artery
  a. cartilage
  a. cartilage graft
  a. nerve
  a. prosthesis
  a. repositioning
auriculomastoid angle
auriculotemporal
  a. artery
  a. nerve
  a. syndrome
auropalpebral
  a. reflex (APR)
Austin Spanish Articulation Test
autism
  infantile a.
  primary a.
  secondary a.
autistic
autoclitic
  a. operant
autogenic
autogenous grafting
autograft
  bone a.

NOTES

autoimmune
    a. disease
    a. inner ear disease
    a. sialoadenitis
    a. sialopathy
autoimmunity
autoinflate
autoinflation
autologous blood
automatic
    a. audiometer
    a. audiometry
    a. gain control
    a. language
    a. speech
    a. volume control (AVC)
automaticity
    auditory-vocal a.
automatism
autonomic
    a. control
    a. nervous system
autophonia
autophony
AUTOVAC autotransfusion system
auxiliary
    modal a.
    a. verb
AVC
    automatic volume control
Avellis syndrome
average
    a. evoked response
      audiometry (AERA)
    pure-tone a. (PTA)

averaging
    signal a.
Avitene
avium
    Mycobacterium a.
AVM
    arteriovenous malformation
avoidance
awareness
    speech a.
axetil
    cefuroxime a.
axial
    a. flap
    a. projection
axillary
    a. artery
    a. vein
axiom
axioversion
axis
    subscapular a.
axon
    a. crossover
axoneme
axonotmesis
azidothymidine (AZT)
AZT
    azidothymidine

B
  B. cell
  B. cell differentiating factor
  B. cell growth factor
  B. cell stimulating factor
  B. lymphocyte
babbling
  non-reduplicated b.
  reduplicated b.
  social b.
Babcock
  Endo-grasper by B.
  B. Endo-grasper
Babinski reflex
baby talk
Bacille bilié de Calmette-Guérin (BCG)
bacillus
  b. Calmette-Guérin (BCG)
  von Frisch b.
bacitracin
  b. irrigation
  b. ointment
back
  b. phoneme
  b. vowel
backbiting forceps
background
  b. artifact
  b. noise
Backhaus towel clip
backing
  b. to velar
backward
  b. coarticulation
  b. masking
backward-biting ostrum punch
bacteria
  aerobic b.
  anaerobic b.
bacterial
  b. infection
  b. sialoadenitis
Bacteroides
  B. melaninogenicus
Bactrim
BADGE
  Bekesy Ascending-Descending
  Gap Evaluation

BAER
  brainstem auditory-evoked
  response
Baillarger's syndrome
Bair Hugger patient warming blanket
Bakamjian flap
Baker self-sumping tube
balance
  Alternate Binaural
  Loudness B. (ABLB)
  Alternate Monaural
  Loudness B. (AMLB)
  b. mechanism
  spatial b.
balanced
  phonetically b. (PB)
baldness
  male-pattern b.
ball forceps
ballistic movement
balloon
  b. occlusion
  b. tamponade
band
  Bünger's b.
  critical b.
  fibrous b.
  b. frequency
  b. spectrum
  synechial b.
  vocal b.
band-pass filter
bandwidth
Bankson Language Screening Test
Banthine
bar
  Bill's b.
  Erich arch b.
  Passavant's b.
Barany
  B. chair
  B. test
barbaralalia
barbiturate
barium
barotrauma
Barrett's ulcer
Barry Five Slate System
Bartholin's duct

basal
- b. age
- b. cell carcinoma
- b. fluency
- b. ganglia
- b. lamella
- b. lamina
- b. pitch
- b. turn cochlea

basaloid
- b. monomorphic adenoma (BMA)
- b. tumor

base
- alar b.
- b. component
- b. rule
- skull b.
- b. structure
- b. word

baseline

basement membrane

basic
- B. Concept Inventory
- B. Language Concepts Test
- b. skill

basilar
- b. artery
- b. artery aneurysm
- b. artery migraine
- b. membrane

basilect

basin
- catch b.

basis
- articulatory b.

basosquamous carcinoma

battery
- Children's Language B.
- Environmental Pre-language B.
- Goldman-Fristoe-Woodcock Auditory Skills B.
- test b.
- vocal capability b.
- Western Aphasia B. (WAB)
- Woodcock Language Proficiency B., English Form

Baumgartner needle holder

Baxter V. Mueller laparoscopic instrumentation

Bayley Scales of Infant Development

bayonet forceps

BC
- bone conduction

BCG
- Bacille bilié de Calmette-Guérin
- bacillus Calmette-Guérin

BCL
- Bekesy comfortable loudness

BD
- behavior disorder
- brain dysfunction

beam
- electron b.
- helium neon b.
- b. splitter

BEAR
- brainstem-evoked auditory response

Bechterew's nucleus

Becker scissors

Bedside Evaluation and Screening Test of Aphasia

behavior
- abusive vocal b.
- adaptive b.
- b. disorder (BD)
- incompatible b.
- b. modification
- operant b.
- social b.
- terminal b.

behavioral
- b. criterion
- b. objective
- b. observation audiometry (BOA)
- b. semantics

behaviorism

Behçet's disease

behind-the-ear (BTE)

Bekesy
- B. Ascending-Descending Gap Evaluation (BADGE)
- B. audiometer
- B. audiometry
- B. comfortable loudness (BCL)
- B. Forward-Reverse Tracing
- B. tracing types

bel

belch

belladonna
 phenobarbital with b.
Bellergal
Bell's
 B. palsy
 B. phenomenon
 B. Visible Speech
bell-shaped curve
Bellugi-Klima's Language
 Comprehension Test
belly
 posterior b.
Bemis suction canister
benign
 b. epithelial neoplasm
 b. intracranial hypertension
 b. intraepithelial
  dyskeratosis
 b. mesenchymal neoplasm
 b. mixed tumor
 b. paroxysmal positional
  vertigo (BPPV)
 b. positional vertigo (BPV)
Benjamin
 B. binocular slimline
  laryngoscope
 B. pediatric operating
  laryngoscope
Benjamin-Havas fiberoptic light
 clip
benzocaine
Benzoin
beriberi
Berko Test
Bernoulli
 B. effect
 B. law
 B. principle
Bernstein test
Berry's ligament
Berry-Talbott Language Test

beta
 b. rhythm
 b. wave
Betadine
bethanechol
 b. chloride
Biaxin
bibliotherapy
BICROS
 bilateral contralateral routing of
  signals
bicuspid tooth
bifid
 b. epiglottis
 b. tongue
bifurcation
bilabial
 b. area
bilateral
 b. abductor paralysis
 b. adductor paralysis
 b. cleft lip
 b. cleft palate
 b. contralateral routing of
  signals (BICROS)
 b. laryngeal paralysis
 b. neck dissection
BiliBlanket phototherapy system
bilingual
 B. Syntax Measure (BSM)
bilingualism
 active b.
 passive b.
Billeau wax curette
Bill's bar
bilobed
 b. flap
 b. transposition flap
bimodal method
binary
 b. principle

NOTES

binaural
   b. CROS
   b. fusion
   b. hearing aid
   b. integration
   b. resynthesis
   b. separation
   b. summation
binder
   Dale abdominal b.
Bing
   B. Test
Bing-Siebenmann malformation
binocular microscopy
biofeedback
   laryngeal image b.
bioflavonoid
Biogel surgeons' gloves
biolinguistic theory
biological act
biologic response modifier
biomodulation
biopsy
   b. forceps
   ultrasound-guided b.
   vertical lip b.
bipartite antrum
bipedicle flap
biphase
   Hall-Morris b.
biphasic stridor
bipolar forceps
birth cry
bisecting
bisensory method
bismuth ingestion
bisyllable
bite
   closed b.
bithermal-caloric test
black
   B. English
   b. hairy tongue
blade
   arrow b.
   lancet b.
   scapular b.
   sickle b.
   b. of the tongue
Blakesley forceps
Blakesley-Weil upturned ethmoid forceps

Blakesley-Wilde forceps
blanket
   Bair Hugger patient warming b.
   mucous b.
blast
   stoma b.
blastomycosis
   laryngeal b.
   South American b.
bleeding
   gastrointestinal b.
   b. tendency
blend
   consonant b.
blending
   auditory b.
   sound b.
bleomycin (BLM)
blephamide
blepharospasm
blindness
   odor b.
   word b.
Blissymbolics
BLM
   bleomycin
block
   clonic b.
   Lell bite b.
   stellate ganglion b.
   tonic b.
blocker
   ganglionic b.
Blom-Singer
   B.-S. tracheoesophageal prosthesis
   B.-S. voice prosthesis
blood
   autologous b.
   b. vessel
blowing
   maximum duration of sustained b.
blowout fracture
blue
   b. mantle
   methylene b.
   b. nevus
   b. sclera
   toluidine b.
blue-lining

blunt lacrimal probe
BMA
  basaloid monomorphic adenoma
BMP
  bone morphogenic protein-2
BOA
  behavioral observation
    audiometry
board
    communication b.
    conversation b.
    direct selection
      communication b.
    encoding communication b.
    scanning communication b.
Bobath method
body
    aortic b.
    asteroid b.
    b. baffle effect
    carotid b.
    foreign b.
    b. hearing aid
    b. language
    b. of the tongue
    tracheobronchial foreign b.
    trapezoid b.
    Verocay b.
Boehm
    B. Test of Basic Concepts-
      Preschool
    B. Test of Basic Concepts-
      R
Boehringer Autovac autotransfusion
  system
Boerhaave syndrome
Boettcher tonsil scissors
bogginess
boilermaker's deafness
bolster

bone
    b. autograft
    b. carpentry
    b. conduction (BC)
    b. conduction level
    corticocancellous b.
    ethmoid b.
    frontal b.
    b. graft
    hyoid b.
    inferior maxillary b.
    inferior turbinated b.
    lacrimal b.
    lateral mastoid b.
    malar b.
    maxillary b.
    medial turbinated b.
    metatarsal b.
    b. morphogenic protein-2
      (BMP)
    nasal b.
    occipital b.
    palatine b.
    parietal b.
    b. sequestrum
    sphenoid b.
    sphenoidal turbinated b.'s
    superior maxillary b.
    superior turbinated b.
    supreme turbinated b.
    temporal b.
    turbinated b.'s
    vaginal process of the
      sphenoid b.
    b. wax
    zygomatic b.
bone-conduction
    b.-c. hearing aid
    b.-c. oscillator
    b.-c. receiver
    b.-c. vibrator

NOTES

bonelet
bony
    b. ankylosis
    b. annulus
    b. atretic plate
    b. labyrinth
    b. plate
    b. protuberance
    b. septum
border
    b. cell
    vermilion b.
Bordetella pertussis
boric acid
Boston
    B. Diagnostic Aphasia
    Examination
    B. University Speech Sound
    Discrimination Test
botulinum toxin
bougie
    Hurst b.
    Jackson steel-stem woven
    filiform b.
    Maloney b.
    Plummer b.
    Tucker b.
bougienage
bound
    b. morpheme
    upper b.
boundary
    language b.
bovine cartilage
bovis
    Actinomyces b.
bowed vocal fold
Bowen-Chalfant Receptive
   Language Inventory
Bowen's disease
bowing
    vocal cord b.
bowl
    mastoid b.
Bowman
    glands of B.
Boyce position
BPPV
   benign paroxysmal positional
    vertigo
BPV
   benign positional vertigo

brace
    CDO orthopedic b.
brachial
    b. fascia
    b. plexus
brachialis muscle
brachioradialis muscle
brachytherapy
bracket
    square b.
bradykinesia
bradykinesthetic
bradylalia
brain
    b. abscess
    b. dysfunction (BD)
    b. mapping
    b. tumor
brainstem
    b. auditory-evoked response
    (BAER)
brainstem-evoked
    b.-e. auditory response
    (BEAR)
    b.-e. response audiometry
    (BSER)
branch
    buccal b.
    cervical b.
    cochlear b.
    facial nerve b.'s
    frontal b.
    zygomatic b.
branches
branchial
    b. arch
    b. cleft cyst
    b. cleft sinus
    b. cyst
    b. fistula
    b. pouch cyst
branching
    b. steps
    b. tree diagram
branchiogenic carcinoma
Branhamella catarrhalis
break
    ascending pitch b.
    descending pitch b.
    phonation b.
    pitch b.
breakdown theory
breast cancer

breath
  b. chewing
  b. stream
Breathe with EEZ
breathiness
breathing
  b. disorder
  donkey b.
  b. method
  opposition b.
Breschet's canal
brief tone audiometry (BTA)
Brigham 1x2 teeth forceps
Briquet's syndrome
Brissaud-Marie syndrome
broad transcription
Broca's
  B. aphasia
  B. area
Brodmann's area 41
Brodmann's area 44
bromide
  methantheline b.
bronchi (*pl. of* bronchus)
bronchial
  b. adenocarcinoma
  b. adenoma
  b. respiration
bronchiectasis
bronchiolar carcinoma
bronchiolitis
bronchitis
  arachidic b.
bronchoesophagology
bronchogenic
  b. carcinoma
  b. cyst
bronchography
bronchopneumonia
bronchoprovocation

bronchoscope
  Holinger b.
bronchoscopic
  b. sponge
  b. sponge carrier
  b. telescope
bronchoscopy
  flexible fiberoptic b.
bronchus, pl. bronchi
Brooke's tumor
brownian
  b. motion
  b. movement
Brown's
  B. sign
  B. test
brow ptosis
Broyle's ligament
brucellosis
Brudzinski's sign
Bruhn method
brushite
bruxism
Bryngelson-Glaspey Test of Articulation
BSER
  brainstem-evoked response audiometry
BSM
  Bilingual Syntax Measure
BTA
  brief tone audiometry
BTE
  behind-the-ear
buccal
  b. branch
  b. cavity
  b. defect
  b. fat
  b. gland
  b. mucosa

NOTES

buccal *(continued)*
    b. mucous gland
    b. muscle
    b. speech
    b. whisper
buccinator
    b. muscle
    b. plication
buccolabial
buccopharyngeal space
buccoversion
Buck wax curette
bud
    taste b.
building
    voice b.
bulb
    jugular b.
    olfactory b.
    saphenous b.
bulbar
    b. paralysis
bulbous internal auditory canal
bulla
    ethmoid b.
    b. ethmoidalis
    frontal b.
bullosa
    concha b.
bullous
    b. myringitis
    b. pemphigoid

bundle
    olivocochlear b.
Bünger's band
bur, burr
    cutting b.
    diamond b.
    Supercut diamond b.
burden
    tumor b.
Burkitt's lymphoma
burn
    chemical b.
    laryngeal b.
    slag b.
    thermal b.
Burow's solution
burr *(var. of* bur)
bursa
    nasopharyngeal b.
    pharyngeal b.
    Thornwaldt b.
burst
    staccato b.
button
    stoma b.
buttonholing
bypass
    colonic b.

C

cathode
celsius
centigrade

CA
chronological age

Ca
cathode

CADL
Communicative Abilities in
Daily Living

CAER
cortical auditory-evoked
response

café
c. au lait spot
c. coronary

Cairns maneuver
calcification
calcitonin
calcium oxalate crystal
calculous disease
calculus
radiopaque c.
salivary c.

Caldwell-Luc
C.-L. incision
C.-L. operation
C.-L. procedure
C.-L. window procedure

Caldwell view
calibrate
calibrated electrical stimulation
calibration overshoot
calibrator
California Consonant Test
calling
word c.

callosal disconnection syndrome
callosum
corpus c.

Calmette-Guérin
Bacille bilié de C.-G.
(BCG)
bacillus C.-G. (BCG)

caloric
c. irrigation
c. nystagmus
C. Test

camera
immersible video c.

CAML
Coarticulation Assessment in
Meaningful Language

camouflage cosmetic
canal
anterior vertical c.
auditory c.
Breschet's c.
bulbous internal auditory c.
c. cap
carotid c.
Dorello's c.
ear c.
external auditory c. (EAC)
facial c.
fallopian c.
c. hearing aid
horizontal c.
c. of Huguier
Huguier's c.
hypoglossal c.
internal auditory c. (IAC)
lateral c.
optic c.
posterior vertical c.
c. resonance response
(CRR)
retrosigmoid/internal
auditory c. (RSG/IAC)
semicircular c.
vestibular c.
vidian c.

canaliculus
c. of chorda tympani
cochlear c.

canalith repositioning procedure
canaloplasty
canal-wall-up technique
cancer
breast c.
glottic c.
head and neck c.
laryngeal c.
oral c.

cancerization
field c.

Candida albicans

candidiasis
    isolated laryngeal c.
canine
    c. fossa
    c. smile
    c. tooth
canister
    Bemis suction c.
    Sep-T-Vac suction c.
Cannon
    white sponge lesion of C.
cannula
    curved c.
    suction c.
cannulation
    duct c.
canthotomy
    lateral c.
canthus
    medial c.
cantilevered bone graft
cap
    canal c.
    c. splint
capacitance
capacitor
capacity
    functional residual c. (FRC)
    inspiratory c. (IC)
    lung c.
    respiratory c.
    total lung c. (TLC)
    vital c. (VC)
capillary hemangioma
capitis (*gen. of* caput)
    anterior rectus c.
    lateral rectus c.
capsule
    otic c.
    parotid c.
    tumor c.
Captopril
caput, gen. **capitis**
    c. angulare of quadratus
    labii superioris
carbamazepine
Carbogen
carbon
    c. dioxide
    c. dioxide laser
carbonization
Carboplatin
carcinogenic

carcinoid
    laryngeal c.
carcinoma
    acinic cell c.
    acinous cell c.
    adenoid cystic c.
    adenoid squamous c.
    adenopapillary c.
    alveolar c.
    basal cell c.
    basosquamous c.
    branchiogenic c.
    bronchiolar c.
    bronchogenic c.
    clear cell c.
    EME c.
      epithelial-myoepithelial
      carcinoma
    epidermoid c.
    epithelial-myoepithelial c.
    (EME carcinoma)
    c. expleomorphic adenoma
    follicular c.
    gastrointestinal c.
    glottic squamous cell c.
    glottic-subglottic squamous
    cell c.
    Hürthle cell c.
    hypopharyngeal squamous
    cell c.
    infraglottic squamous cell c.
    keratinizing squamous
    cell c.
    laryngeal c.
    lobular c.
    Merkel cell c.
    microcystic adnexal c.
    morpheaform basal cell c.
    mucoepidermoid c.
    mucus-producing
    adenopapillary c.
    nasopharyngeal c.
    oat cell c.
    pancreatic c.
    parotid c.
    postcricoid c.
    postcricoid squamous cell c.
    pseudosarcomatous c.
    recurrent squamous cell c.
    renal cell c.
    salivary duct c. (SDC)
    sebaceous c.
    small cell c.

spindle cell c.
squamous cell c. (SCC)
subglottic squamous cell c.
supraglottic squamous
  cell c.
terminal duct c.
transglottic squamous cell c.
transitional cell c.
undifferentiated c.
unresectable squamous
  cell c.
verrucous c.

card

Speech Improvement C.'s

**cardiac-evoked response audiometry
  (CERA)**
cardiac gland
cardinal vowel
cardiovascular disease
care

palliative c.
wound c.

Cargot ear
Carhart notch
caries
carina
carinii

Pneumocystis c.

Carlen's mediastinoscope
C-arm

Siremobil C.-a. unit

carmustine
caroticotympanic artery
carotid

c. air cell
c. aneurysm
c. artery
c. body
c. canal
c. sheath

carpentry

bone c.

Carrell Discrimination Test
carrier

bronchoscopic sponge c.
c. phrase

Carrow

C. Auditory-Visual Abilities
  Test
C. Elicited Language
  Inventory (CELI)

carryover
cartilage

alar c.
arytenoid c.
auricular c.
bovine c.
conchal c.
corniculate c.
costal c.
cricoid c.
cuneiform c.
c. graft
hyoid c.
laryngeal c.
lateral c.
lower lateral c.
quadrangular c.
septal c.
thyroid c.
tragal c.
upper lateral c.
upper lateral nasal c.
vomeronasal c.
Wrisberg's c.

cartilago triticea
cascade

clotting c.

case

accusative c.
genitive c.

NOTES

29

case *(continued)*
    c. grammar
    nominative c.
    objective c.
    possessive c.
    c. relations
    subjective c.
caseosa
    coryza c.
    ozena c.
    rhinitis c.
caseous purulent rhinorrhea
CAT
    computerized axial tomography
    CAT scan
cat
    c. cry syndrome
    c. scratch disease
catalase
catalogia
catarrh
    tubal c.
catarrhal
    c. deafness
    c. disease
    c. otitis media
catarrhalis
    Branhamella c.
    Neisseria c.
catastrophic response
catch
    c. basin
    glottal c.
category
    grammatical c.
    lexical c.
catenative
catheter
    ARROWgard central
      venous c.
    Fogarty adherent clot c.
    transoral c.
catheterization
cathode (C, Ca)
Cattel Scale
cauda helicis
caudal
cauliflower ear
causality
caustic
    acid c.
    alkali c.
    c. ingestion

cave
    Meckel's c.
cavernous
    c. hemangioma
    c. lymphangiohemangioma
    c. sinus
    c. sinus thrombosis
cavity
    buccal c.
    mastoid c.
    nasal c.
    nonseptate c.
    oral c.
    tympanic c.
    vitreous c.
cavum conchae
Cawthorne-Day procedure
CCL cell
CCNU
    cyclohexylchloroethylnitrosurea
    lomustine
CDDP
    cisplatin
CDO orthopedic brace
cecum
    foramen c.
    vestibular c.
cefixime
cefpodoxime proxetil
cefuroxime
    c. axetil
    c. sodium
CELF
    Clinical Evaluation of Language
    Functions
CELI
    Carrow Elicited Language
    Inventory
cell
    acinar c.
    agger nasi c.
    air c.
    angulated c.
    anterior ethmoidal air c.
    antigen-presenting c.
    antral c.
    apical c.
    B c.
    border c.
    carotid air c.
    CCL c.
      centrocyte-like cell
    centrocyte-like c. (CCL cell)

chondroid c.
ciliated c.
c.'s of Claudius
cochlear hair c.
c. cycle
dendritic c.
epitympanic air c.
ethmoid c.
ethmoidal c.
ethmoidal labyrinth c.
follicular dendritic c. (FDC)
frontoethmoidal c.
giant c.
goblet c.
hair c.
Haller's c.
c.'s of Hansen
helper-inducer T c.
helper T c.
hyaline c.
inflammatory c.
infundibular c.
interdigitating dendritic c.
  (IDC)
killer c.
Langerhans' c.'s
Langhans' c.'s
lymphokine-activated
  killer c. (LAK)
macular hair c.
mast c.
mastoid tip c.
microvillar c.
Mikulicz c.
monocytoid c.
mucus-secreting c.
natural killer c.'s (NK)
nerve c.
olfactory c.
oncocytic epithelial c.
onodi c.

plasma c.
postcarotid air c.
posterior ethmoidal c.
precarotid air c.
precochlear c.
Reed-Sternberg c.
retrofacial c.
Schwann c.
serous c.
sinus group of air c.
spindle c.
subtubal air c.
suppressor-effector T c.
suppressor-inducer T c.
suppressor T c.
supracarotid air c.
supracochlear air c.
supraorbital air c.
sustentacular c.
T c.
tympanic c.
zygomal c.
cell-mediated immunity
cellular pleomorphism
cellulitis
orbital c.
periorbital c.
peritonsillar c.
preseptal c.
celsius (C)
center
germinal c.
language c.
center-action forceps
centigrade (C)
central
c. aphasia
c. auditory abilities
c. auditory disorder
c. auditory function
c. auditory perception

NOTES

31

central *(continued)*
   c. auditory process
   c. deafness
   c. hearing
   c. hearing loss
   c. incisor tooth
   c. language disorder (CLD)
   c. language imbalance
   c. masking
   c. nervous system (CNS)
   c. speech range
   c. sulcus
   c. tendency
   c. vowel
centration
centrocyte-like cell (CCL cell)
cephalgia
   Horton's histamine c.
cephalic
cephalicus
   herpes zoster c.
CERA
   cardiac-evoked response
   audiometry
cerebellar
   c. abscess
   c. vein
cerebellopontine (CP)
   c. angle (CPA)
   c. angle tumor
cerebellum
   flocculus of c.
cerebral
   c. anoxia
   c. aqueduct
   c. cortex
   c. dominance
   c. dominance and
   handedness theory
   c. edema
   c. localization
   c. palsy
   c. palsy symptomatology
   c. thumb
   zero c.
cerebri
   falx c.
   pseudotumor c.
cerebropalatine angle
cerebrospinal
   c. fluid (CSF)

   c. fluid leak
   c. fluid rhinorrhea
cerebrovascular accident (CVA)
cerebrum
cerumen
   impacted c.
ceruminoma
cervical
   c. branch
   c. esophagus
   c. fascia
   c. flap
   c. ganglion
   c. metastasis
   c. muscle contraction
   c. plexus
   c. skin replacement
   c. soft tissue
   c. sympathectomy
   c. sympathetic nerve
   c. vertigo
cervicofacial trunk
cervicomastoid region
cervix
CFM
   chemotactic factor for
   macrophage
Chagas-Cruz disease
Chagas' disease
chain
   ossicle c.
   ossicular c.
   polypeptide c.
chaining
chair
   Barany c.
   computerized rotary c.
   Video-fluoroscopic
   imaging c.
chamber
   anechoic c.
   echo c.
   no-echo c.
change
   phylogentic c.
character
characteristic
   sexual c.'s
charts
   Northampton c.
Chausse
   third projection of C.

cheek
    c. advancement flap
    c. flap
    c. rotation flap
    c. tone
cheilitis
    granulomatous c.
chemical
    c. burn
    c. shift
chemodectoma
chemoreceptor
chemotactic factor for macrophage (CFM)
chemotherapy
    adjuvant c.
    combination c.
    intra-arterial c.
    neoadjuvant c.
cherry hemangioma
chest
    c. pulse
    c. voice
chewing
    breath c.
    c. method
CHI
    closed head injury
chiasm
    optic c.
chickenpox
Chick patient transfer device
childhood
    c. aphasia
    c. schizophrenia
children
    Kaufman Assessment Battery for C.
    Porch Index of Communicative Abilities in C. (PICAC)

    Short Test for Use with Cerebral Palsy C.
    Test of Language Competence for C. (TLC-C)
    Token Test for C.
    Wechsler Intelligence Scale for C.-Revised (WISC-R)
Children's
    C. Language Battery
    C. Language Processes
chiloschisis
chink
    glottal c.
chin-nose view
chin spasm
Chlamydia trachomatis
chlorambucil
chloramphenicol
chloride
    bethanechol c.
    edrophonium c.
Chloromycetin
chlortetracycline
    c. ointment
choana, pl. choanae
choanal
    c. atresia
    c. opening
cholangiography
cholangiopancreatography
    endoscopic c.
cholesteatoma
    acquired c.
    attic c.
    congenital c.
    iatrogenic c.
    c. pearl
    rhinitis c.
cholesterol
    c. crystal

NOTES

cholesterol *(continued)*
 c. granuloma
 c. granuloma cyst
cholinergic
chondritis
chondrogenic sarcoma
chondroid cell
chondroma
 laryngeal c.
 tracheal c.
chondrosarcoma
 extraosseous c.
choral
 c. reading
 c. speaking
chorda
 c. tympani
 c. tympani nerve
chorditis
chordoma
chorea
choreoathetosis
choriomeningitis
 lymphocytic c.
choristoma
chromation
 nuclear c.
chromic suture
chromosome 21-trisomy syndrome
chronaxie
chronic
 c. active hepatitis
 c. cicatricial laryngeal
  stenosis
 c. diffuse external otitis
 c. ethmoiditis
 c. fatigue syndrome
 c. fibrotic tonsillitis
 c. frontal sinusitis
 c. hypertrophic
  rhinosinusitis
 c. laryngitis
 c. maxillary sinusitis
 c. mononucleosis syndrome
 c. rhinitis
 c. sialadenitis
 c. stenosing external otitis
 c. suppurative otitis media
chronological age (CA)
chunking
chyle
 c. fistula
 c. leak

cicatrization
 epithelial c.
cilia (*pl. of* cilium)
ciliary motion
ciliated cell
cilium, pl. cilia
 olfactory c.
 respiratory c.
cine-esophagogram
cinefluorography
cinefluoroscopy
cineradiography
cineroentgenography
ciprofloxacin
circle of Willis
circuit
 convergence c.
 divergence c.
 feedback reduction c. (FRC)
 neuronal c.
 telephone booster c.
circulation
 cutaneous c.
circumaural
 c. hearing protection device
circumferential esophageal
 reconstruction
circumflex
 c. iliac artery
 c. scapular artery
 c. scapular pedicle
 c. scapular vessel
circumlocution
circumscribed labyrinthitis
cirrhosis
 Laennec's c.
cisplatin (CDDP)
cis-retinoic acid
cistern
clamp
 Cottle columella c.
clarithromycin
Clark-Madison Test of Oral
 Language
Clark Picture Phonetic Inventory
class
 closed c.
 open c.
 word c.
 c. word
classical conditioning
classification
 Angle's c.

c. of cleft palate
House-Brackmann c.
Seddon c.
sentence c.
Sunderland's c.
tongue thrust c.
tympanogram c. (Feldman model)
tympanogram c. (Jerger model)
Claudius
cells of C.
clause
constituent c.
dependent c.
embedded c.
independent c.
main c.
principal c.
subordinate c.
c. terminal
clavicular
CLD
central language disorder
clear cell carcinoma
cleavage plane
cleft
atypical c.
labial c.
laryngeal c.
laryngotracheoesophageal c.
c. lip
nose c.
c. palate
palatomaxillary c.
rare c.
soft palate c.
tracheoesophageal c.
Clerf-Arrowsmith safety pin closer
click
glottal c.

clindamycin
clinical
c. audiology
C. Evaluation of Language Functions (CELF)
C. Probes of Articulation Consistency (C-PAC)
clinician
language c.
speech and language c.
voice c.
clinoid process
clip
Backhaus towel c.
Benjamin-Havas fiberoptic light c.
Raney c.
Zimmer c.
clipped word
clipping
peak c.
clivus
C. L. Jackson
C. L. Jackson head-holding forceps
C. L. Jackson pin-bending costophrenic forceps
clonal proliferation
clonic
c. block
clonus
close
c. transcription
c. vowel
closed
c. bite
C. Chain Exercise Attachment
c. class
c. head injury (CHI)

NOTES

closed *(continued)*
    c. juncture
    c. syllable
closer
    Clerf-Arrowsmith safety
      pin c.
closure
    auditory c.
    floor-of-mouth c.
    glottic c.
    grammatic c.
    SutureStrip Plus wound c.
    velopharyngeal c.
    visual c.
    watertight c.
clot
clotting
    c. abnormality
    c. cascade
Club
    Lost Cord C.
    Nu Voice C.
cluster
    consonant c.
    c. headache
    c. reduction
    reduction of c.'s
cluttering
CMV
    cytomegalovirus
CNS
    central nervous system
CNT
    could not test
CO2 laser
coagulation
    laser c.
Coakley tenaculum
coalescence
coalescent mastoiditis
coarticulation
    anticipatory c.
    C. Assessment in
      Meaningful Language
      (CAML)
    backward c.
    forward c.
coat
    fuzzy c.
    mucosal c.
cobra-head drill
cocaine
    c. anesthesia

coccidioidomycosis
cochlea
    basal turn c.
cochlear
    c. aplasia
    c. aqueduct
    c. artery
    c. branch
    c. canaliculus
    c. duct
    c. echo
    c. hair cell
    c. hydrops
    c. microphonic
    c. nerve
    c. nucleus
    c. partition
    c. reflex
    c. reserve
    c. stereocilia
    c. tuning
    c. vein
    c. window
cochleariform process
cochleo-orbicular
    c.-o. reflex
cochleopalpebral
    c. reflex (CPR)
cochleosacculotomy
cochleostomy
cochleovestibular
    c. approach
    c. neurectomy (CVN)
coefficient
    alternate forms reliability c.
    comparable forms
      reliability c.
    c. of correlation
    reliability c.
    test-retest reliability c.
cognate
    c. confusion
cognition
cognitive
    c. development
    c. development stage
    c. dissonance
    c. distancing
    c. mapping
    c. style
cohesive device
coil
    induction c.

cold
common c.
c. light
cold-running
c.-r. speech
C.-r. Speech Test
coli
Escherichia c.
Colin STBP-780 stress test blood pressure monitor
colistimethate
colistin
collagen
c. antibody
c. injection
microfibrillar c.
collagenous tissue
collagen-vascular disease
collapse
inspiratory laryngeal c.
collar
shower c.
collection
globular c.
saccular c.
collective monologue
collector
parotid c.
Collet-Sicard syndrome
colliculus
inferior c.
Collis gastroplasty
colloquial
colloquialism
colonic bypass
colony-stimulating factor (CSF)
color-flow Doppler
Coloured Progressive Matrices
Columbia Mental Maturity Scale
columella, pl. columellae

columellar
c. reconstruction
c. repair
columnar
combination chemotherapy
combined method
comedocarcinoma
comitantes
venae c.
commando procedure
commissural inhibition
commissure
anterior c.
common
c. carotid artery
c. cold
c. facial vein
commune
crus c.
communication
C. Abilities Diagnostic Test and Screen
aided augmentative c.
alternative c.
augmentative c.
c. board
c. disorder
Evaluating Acquired Skills in C. (EASIC)
c. failure theory
nonoral c.
nonvocal c.
oral c.
c. science
C. Screen
total c.
unaided augmentative c.
communicative
C. Abilities in Daily Living (CADL)
c. competence

NOTES

communicative *(continued)*
    c. disorder
    c. interaction
    c. technique
communicologist
communicology
community
    dialect speech c.
    speech c.
compact phoneme
comparable forms reliability
    coefficient
comparative
    c. linguistics
    c. research
COMPAT enteral feeding pump
Compazine
compensation
    worker's c.
compensatory movement
competence
    communicative c.
    Evaluating
       Communicative C.
    Fisher-Logemann Test of
       Articulation C.
    linguistic c.
    Test of Language C. (TLC)
    Tests of Minimal
       Articulation C.
    velopharyngeal c.
competing
    c. messages
    c. messages integration
    C. Sentence Test
complement
    objective c.
    c. system
complemental air
complementary distribution
complete
    c. cleft palate
    c. recruitment
Completing Sentence Test (CST)
completion thyroidectomy
complex
    AIDS-related c. (ARC)
    immune c.
    major histocompatibility c.
    (MHC)
    c. noise
    olivary c.
    c. sentence

sicca c.
C. Speech Sound
    Discrimination Test
superior olivary c.
    c. syllabic
    c. tone
    c. wave
    c. word
compliance
complication
component
    base c.
    grammatical c.
    linguistic c.
    morphophonemic c.
    secretory c.
composite
    c. flap
    c. resection
compound
    c. consonant
    c. flap
    N-nitroso c.
    nominal c.
    c. sentence
    c. word
compound-complex sentence
comprehension
    Assessment of Children's
       Language C. (ACLC)
    c. span
compressed speech
compression
    c. amplification
    c. bone conduction
    esophageal c.
    c. hearing aid
    nerve c.
    neurovascular cross c.
    (NVCC)
    c. plating
    c. switch
    tracheal c.
    variable release c.
Compton-Hutton Phonological
    Assessment
Compton Speech and Language
    Screening Evaluation
compulsion
computed tomography (CT)
computerized
    c. axial tomography (CAT)
    c. rotary chair

computer language
concatenation
concept
    Boehm Test of Basic C.'s-
      Preschool
    Boehm Test of Basic C.'s-R
    critical band c.
    object c.
    self-role c.
Concept CTS Relief Kit for carpal
  tunnel release
conceptual disorder
conceptualization
concha, pl. conchae
    c. bullosa
    cavum conchae
    cymba conchae
    inferior c.
    inferior nasal c.
    medial nasal c.
    nasal conchae
    sphenoidal nasal conchae
    superior nasal c.
    supreme nasal c.
conchal
    c. cartilage
    c. crest of maxilla
concrete operations period
concretism
concurrent validity
concussion
condensation
condenser
condition
conditioned
    c. disintegration theory
    c. orientation reflex
      audiometry (COR)
    c. reinforcer
    c. response
    c. stimulus

conditioning
    classical c.
    counter c.
    instrumental c.
    operant c.
    phonological c.
    respondent c.
    tangible reinforcement of
      operant c.
conductance
conduction
    air c. (AC)
    c. aphasia
    bone c. (BC)
    compression bone c.
    distortional bone c.
    inertial bond c.
    osteotympanic bone c.
    sensory acuity level bone c.
conductive
    c. deafness
    c. hearing loss
conductivity
condylar emissary vein
cone
    intraoral c.
    c. of light
conference
    Hearing Aid Industry C.
      (HAIC)
configuration
    audiogram c.
    word c.
confused language
confusion
    cognate c.
congenita
    dyskeratosis c.
    pachyonychia c.
congenital
    c. cholesteatoma

NOTES

congenital *(continued)*
    c. deafness
    c. dysosmia
    c. luetic labyrinthitis
    c. malformation
    c. polycystic disease
    c. subglottic hemangioma
congestion
    nasal c.
coniotomy
conjoiner
conjunction
Conley incision
connected speech
connection
    vestibulocerebellar c.
connective
    c. tissue
    c. tissue graft
connector
    Y-port c.
connotation
consent
    informed c.
consequence
conservation
    hearing c.
    speech c.
    c. surgery
consistency
    Clinical Probes of
      Articulation C. (C-PAC)
    c. effect
    object c.
    perceptual c.
consonance
consonant
    abutting c.
    arresting c.
    c. blend
    c. cluster
    compound c.
    deletion of final c.
    deletion of initial c.
    devoicing of final c.
    double c.
    flap c.
    fortis c.
    lax c.
    lenis c.
    nasal c.
    c. position

    prevocalic voicing of c.
    releasing c.
    velarized c.
    vibrant c.
    voiced c.
    voiceless c.
    c. voicing
    c.-vowel (CV)
    c.-vowel-consonant (CVC)
consonantal
consonant-injection method
consonant-vowel preference
constancy
constituent
    c. clause
    immediate sentence c.
    sentence c.
    c. sentence
constraint
    semantic c.
constricted vocal production
constriction
    nares c.
    vocal c.
constrictor
    inferior pharyngeal c.
    middle pharyngeal c.
    c. pharyngeal muscle
    superior pharyngeal c.
construction
    absolute c.
    endocentric c.
    exocentric c.
constructional apraxia
construct validity
contact
    c. allergic stomatitis
    c. dermatitis
    c. granuloma
    c. lens
    c. ulcer
content
    language c.
    c. validity
    c. word
contentive word
context
    phonetic c.
contiguity disorder
contingency management
contingent
continuant

continuous
    c. positive airway pressure
      (CPAP)
    c. reinforcement schedule
contour
    c. defect
    equal loudness c.
    intonation c.
    c. restoration
    terminal c.
contraction
    cervical muscle c.
    false muscle c.
    muscle c.
    stapes tendon c.
contracture
contraindication
contralateral
    c. routing of signals
      (CROS)
contrast
    air-iodinated c.
    maximal c.
    minimal c.
    c. study
contrastive
    c. distribution
    c. linguistics
control
    acoustic gain c.
    automatic gain c.
    automatic volume c. (AVC)
    autonomic c.
    gain c.
    c. group
    humoral c.
    manual volume c.
    rate c.
    resonant peak c.
    tone c.
    volume c.

conus elasticus
convergence circuit
conversational postulates
conversation board
Converse
    scalping flap of C.
conversion
    c. aphonia
    c. deafness
    c. hysteria
    c. reaction
convoluted
convolution
convulsion
cooing
Cool Comfort cold pack
coordination
    visual-motor c.
coprolalia
copula
COR
    conditioned orientation reflex
      audiometry
cord
    false vocal c.
    vocal c.
cordectomy
core vocabulary
corkscrew esophagus
corneal ulceration
corneoretinal potential
corner-of-the-mouth smile
corniculate
    c. cartilage
coronal
    c. oblique projection
    c. plane
    c. projection
coronary
    c. artery disease

NOTES

coronary *(continued)*
café c.
c. thrombosis
coronoidectomy
coronoid process
cor pulmonale
corpus, pl. **corpora**
c. callosum
correction
speech c.
correctionist
speech c.
corrective
c. feedback
c. therapy (CT)
correlation
coefficient of c.
negative c.
Pearson product-moment coefficient of c.
positive c.
corrugator
c. muscle
c. supercilia muscle
cortex, pl. **cortices**
auditory c.
cerebral c.
mastoid c.
Corti
organ of C.
tunnel of C.
cortical
c. auditory-evoked response (CAER)
c. deafness
c. lateralization
c. respiration
c. vein
cortices (*pl. of* cortex)
corticocancellous bone
corticosteroid
17-hydroxy c.
cortilymph
cortisol
Corynebacterium
C. diphtheriae
C. hemolyticum
coryza
c. caseosa
cosine wave
cosmesis
cosmetic
camouflage c.

costal
c. cartilage
c. cartilage graft
Costen's syndrome
Cottle
C. columella clamp
C. elevator
C. knife
C. nasal speculum
cottonoid
cotton pledget
Cotunnius
nerve of C.
cough
nervous c.
spasmodic laryngeal c.
could not test (CNT)
coulomb (Q)
counseling
count
helper T-cell c.
T-cell c.
word c.
counter conditioning
coup de glotte
coupler
coupling
nasal c.
covert response
Coxsackievirus
CP
cerebellopontine
CPA
cerebellopontine angle
C-PAC
Clinical Probes of Articulation Consistency
CPAP
continuous positive airway pressure
CPR
cochleopalpebral reflex
CPS
cycles per second
cradle
neonatal auditory response c.
cramp
laryngeal c.
cranial
c. base defect
c. fossa defect

c. nerve
c. polyneuritis
craniofacial
c. anomaly
c. disjunction
c. resection
craniopharyngioma
craniotomy
cream
Silvadene c.
crease
lateral neck c.
preauricular c.
crest
ampullary c.
falciform c.
iliac c.
vertical c.
cretinism
Crib-O-Gram
cribriform plate
cribrosa
lamina c.
cricoarytenoid
c. ankylosis
c. arthrodesis
c. joint
c. muscle
cricoid
c. cartilage
cricopharyngeal myotomy
cricopharyngeus muscle
cricothyroid
c. angle
c. artery
c. joint
c. membrane
c. muscle
cricothyroidotomy
cricothyrotomy
cricovocal membrane

cri du chat syndrome
cris-CROS
crista
c. ampullaris
c. falciformis
c. galli
criterion, pl. criteria
behavioral c.
c. related validity
criterion-referenced test
critical
c. band
c. band concept
crocodile tears
Crohn's disease
cromolyn sodium
CROS
contralateral routing of signals
binaural CROS
power CROS
crossbar
cross-bite
cross-consonant injection method
crossed laterality
cross-facial
c.-f. nerve graft
c.-f. technique
cross hearing
cross-modality perception
crossover
axon c.
facial nerve c.
cross-talk
croup
inflammatory c.
spasmodic c.
c. tent
CRR
canal resonance response
cruciate incision

NOTES

crura
crus, pl. **crura**
    c. commune
    lateral c.
    posterior c.
cry
    birth c.
cryoglobulin
cryosurgery
cryptococcal meningitis
crystal
    calcium oxalate c.
    cholesterol c.
    tyrosine c.
CSF
    cerebrospinal fluid
    colony-stimulating factor
CST
    Completing Sentence Test
CT
    computed tomography
    corrective therapy
CTX
    cyclophosphamide
cubital artery
cuboidal
cue
    auditory c.
    kinesthetic c.
    visual c.
cued speech
cuff
    V-Lok disposable blood
      pressure c.
cuirass ventilation
cul-de-sac
cultural norm
Culture Fair Intelligence Test
cuneiform
    c. cartilage
    c. cartilage of Wrisberg
cupped forceps
cupula
cupulolithiasis
cupulometry
curettage
curette, curet
    Billeau wax c.
    Buck wax c.
    disposable c.
    oval c.
    Shapleigh wax c.

    sharp loop c.
    wax c.
current
    alternating c. (AC)
    direct c. (DC)
curse
    Ondine's c.
curve
    articulation c.
    bell-shaped c.
    dipper c.
    discrimination c.
    falling c.
    frequency response c.
    gaussian c.
    isodose c.
    marked falling c.
    normal c.
    normal probability c.
    probability c.
    saddle c.
    saucer c.
    shadow c.
    sharply falling c.
    ski slope c.
    steep drop c.
    strength duration c.
    sudden drop c.
    trough c.
    tuning c.
    U-shaped c.
    waterfall c.
curved
    c. cannula
    c. scissors
    c. turbinate scissors
    c. turbinectomy scissors
curvilinear incision
CUSA laparoscopic tip
Cushing
    C. forceps
    C. syndrome
    C. ulcer
cushion
    Passavant's c.
cusp
cuspid tooth
cut
    full spectrum low c.
cutaneous
    c. circulation
    c. flap
    c. forearm flap

c. horn
c. paddle
cutting bur
CV
consonant-vowel
CVA
cerebrovascular accident
CVC
consonant-vowel-consonant
CVN
cochleovestibular neurectomy
cyanosis
cybernetics
cybernetic theory of stuttering
cycle
cell c.
duty c.
glottal c.
vibratory c.
cycles per second (CPS)
cyclohexylchloroethylnitrosurea (CCNU)
cyclophosphamide (CTX)
cylindroma
cylindromatous lesion
cymba conchae
cyst
arachnoid c.
branchial c.
branchial cleft c.
branchial pouch c.
bronchogenic c.
cholesterol granuloma c.
dentigerous c.
dermoid c.
enteric c.
enterogenous c.
epidermoid c.
follicular c.
globulomaxillary c.
incisive canal c.

laryngeal saccular c.
lymphoepithelial c.
mandibular c.
maxillary c.
maxillary sinus c.
mucosal c.
mucous c.
mucous retention c.
nasopalatine duct c.
nasopharyngeal c.
nonsecreting mucosal c.
papillary c.
periosteal c.
pilar c.
preauricular c.
radicular c.
retention c.
root c.
saccular c.
salivary duct c.
sebaceous c.
sphenoidal c.
teratoid c.
Thornwaldt c.
thyroglossal c.
thyroglossal duct c.
cystic
c. adenoid epithelioma
c. fibrosis
c. hygroma
c. lymphoepithelial AIDS-related lesion
c. oncocytic metaplasia
cysticum
epithelioma adenoides c.
cytology
aspiration biopsy c.
needle aspiration c.
cytomegalic inclusion disease
cytomegalovirus (CMV)

NOTES

cytoplasm
   oxyphilic c.
cytoplasmic eosinophilia
cytosine
   c. arabinosyl

cytotoxicity
   antibody-dependent cellular c. (ADCC)

dacarbazine (DTIC)
dacryocystorhinostomy (DCR)
dacryorhinocystostomy
dactyl
    d. speech
dactylology
D.A.D. mattress
DAF
    delayed auditory feedback
Dale
    D. abdominal binder
    D. Foley catheter holder
    D. oxygen cannula support
    D. tracheostomy tube
      holder
    D. ventilator tubing support
damage
    noise-induced d.
damped wave
damping
DAPS
    Differentiation of Auditory
    Perception Skill
dapsone
dark lateral
Darwin's tubercle
DASE
    Denver Articulation Screening
    Examination
DAT
    Developmental Articulation Test
Datascope pulse oximeter
dative
daunorubicin
Davis-Kitlowski procedure
Davol dermatome
dB
    decibel
DC
    direct current
DCR
    dacryocystorhinostomy
dead room
deaf
    d. mute
    d. speech
deaffrication
deafness
    adventitious d.
    boilermaker's d.

    catarrhal d.
    central d.
    conductive d.
    congenital d.
    conversion d.
    cortical d.
    familial d.
    functional d.
    high frequency d.
    hysterical d.
    industrial d.
    mixed d.
    nerve d.
    noise-induced d.
    nonorganic d.
    occupational d.
    postlingual d.
    prelingual d.
    prevocational d.
    psychogenic d.
    pure word d.
    sensorineural d.
    tone d.
    toxic d.
    word d.
Dean
    D. periosteal elevator
    D. tonsil hemostat
debulking
decannulation
decay
    acoustic reflex d.
    free induction d. (FID)
    d. period
    d. rate
    rate of d.
    tone d.
decentration
decibel (dB)
deciduous tooth
declarative sentence
decoder
decoding
decompression
    facial nerve d.
    gastric d.
    microvascular d. (MVD)
    orbital d.
deconditioning

decongestant
    topical d.
decongestion
    local d.
decruitment
decussation
Dedo laryngoscope
deduction
deep
    d. articulation test
    d. petrosal nerve
    d. structure
    D. Test of Articulation
de-epithelialization
deep-lobe tumor
defatting
defect
    buccal d.
    contour d.
    cranial base d.
    cranial fossa d.
    intraoral mucosal d.
    orbitomaxillary d.
    postresection d.
    saddle-nose d.
    segmental bone d.
    speech d.
deficiency
    American Association On
      Mental D. (AAMD)
    iron d.
    vitamin d.
    vitamin A d.
    vitamin B d.
defined frequency
deformity
    Andy Gump d.
    facial d.
    Mondini d.
degeneration
    Wallerian d.
deglutition
degrees
    hearing impairment d.
dehiscence
    intimal d.
dehydroepiandrosterone
dehydrogenase
    11β-hydroxysteroid d.
    lactic d.
    malic d.
dehydrosterone
deictic

Deiters' nucleus
deixis
déjà vu
Déjérine syndrome
delayed
    d. auditory feedback (DAF)
    d. echolalia
    d. feedback audiometry
      (DFA)
    d. language
    d. reinforcer
    d. response
    d. speech
deletion
    d. of final consonant
    d. of initial consonant
    stridency d.
    syllable d.
    d. of unstressed syllable
    unstressed syllable d.
    weak syllable d.
delphian node
Del Rio Language Screening Test,
    English/Spanish
delta
    d. rhythm
    d. wave
deltopectoral flap
deltoscapular flap
demarcation
dementia
Demerol
Demodex folliculorum
demonstrative
demonstrative-entity
De Morgan spot
denasal
denasality
denasalization
denaturation
dendrite
dendritic cell
denervated muscle
Dennis Browne tonsil forceps
denotation
densitometry
density
    sound power d.
dental
    d. amalgam
    d. arch
    d. lisp
    d. occlusion

d. restoration
d. trauma
dentate
dentigerous cyst
dentition
  prosthetic d.
denude
Denver Articulation Screening Examination (DASE)
depalatalization
dependent clause
depletion
  end-stage nutritional d.
depressor
  d. anguli oris muscle
  d. muscle
  d. septi
de Quervain's granulomatous thyroiditis
derivation
  sentence d.
  d. of a sentence
derived sentence
dermabrasion
dermal
  d. analogue tumor
  d. fat free flap
  d. fat free tissue transfer
  d. fat pedicles flap
  d. pouch
  d. pouch reconstruction
dermatitis
  atopic d.
  contact d.
  d. herpetiformis
  d. medicamentosa
  seborrheic d.
  d. venenata
dermatome
  Davol d.

dermatomyositis
dermatosis papulosa nigra
dermoid cyst
descending
  d. palatine artery
  d. pitch break
  d. technique
  d. vestibular nucleus
descriptive phonetics
desensitization
desiccation
desk-type auditory trainer
desmosome
desquamating epithelium
desquamation
Detachol
detectability threshold
detection
  gap d.
  speech d.
  d. threshold
determiner
  regular d.
determinism
  linguistic d.
development
  Bayley Scales of Infant D.
  cognitive d.
  Houston Test for Language D.
  language d.
  Screening Kit of Language D. (SKOLD)
  Sequenced Inventory of Communication D.
  speech d.
  Test of Language D.-Intermediate (TOLD-I)
  Test of Language D.-Primary (TOLD-P)

NOTES

development *(continued)*
Tests of Early Language D.
(TELD)
Utah Test of Language D.
developmental
d. age
d. aphasia
D. Articulation Test (DAT)
d. period
d. phonological process
d. scale
D. Sentence Scoring (DSS)
deviant
d. articulation
d. language
d. speech
d. swallowing
deviated septum
deviation
standard d.
device
Chick patient transfer d.
circumaural hearing
protection d.
cohesive d.
hearing protection d. (HPD)
insert hearing protection d.
Insta-Mold ear protection d.
interrupter d.
language acquisition d.
(LAD)
presyntactic d.
semiaural hearing
protection d.
devoicing of final consonant
dewlap
radiation d.
dexamethasone
dexterity
dextral
dextrality
Dextran
dextromethorphan
DFA
delayed feedback audiometry
diabetes mellitus
diabetic neuropathy
diacritic
diadochokinesis
diagnosis
differential d.
diagnosogenic theory

diagnostic
d. articulation test
d. audiology
d. audiometry
d. teaching
d. test
d. therapy (Dx)
diagram
branching tree d.
tree d.
dialect
regional d.
d. speech community
diameter
aerodynamic equivalent d.
(AED)
internal d.
diamond
d. bur
Diamox
diaphragm
styloid d.
diaphragmatic-abdominal respiration
diaphragmatic hernia
diathermal needle
diathesis
diazepam
Dibromodulcitol
dichotic
D. Consonant-Vowel Test
D. Digits
d. listening
d. messages
dichotomous
dichotomy
diction
dielectric
diencephalon
diethyldithiocarbamate
sodium d.
difference
just noticeable d. (JND)
language d.
d. limen (DL)
masking level d.
d. tone
differential
d. diagnosis
d. function
d. reinforcement
d. relaxation
d. response
d. threshold

differentiation
  auditory d.
  D. of Auditory Perception Skill (DAPS)
diffracted wave
diffuse
  d. esophageal spasm
  d. hyperplasia
  d. large cell lymphoma
  d. phoneme
  d. serous labyrinthitis
  d. suppurative labyrinthitis
  d. vocal polyposis
digastric
  d. fossa
  d. muscle
  d. muscle flap
  d. ridge
digital
  d. hearing aid
  d. manipulation
digits
  Dichotic D.
diglossia
digraph
Dilantin
dilatans
  pneumosinus d.
dilatation
  esophageal d.
dilator
  Jackson triangular brass d.
  d. naris
  d. naris muscle
  tracheoesophageal puncture d.
dimethyltrianzeno-imidazole-carboxamide (DTIC)
diminutive
Dinamap Plus multiparameter monitor

diode
diotic
  d. listening
  d. messages
dioxide
  carbon d.
  sulfur d. (SO₂)
diphasic spike
diphemanil methylsulfate
diphenylhydantoin
diphtheria
diphtheriae
  Corynebacterium d.
diphthong
diplacusis
diplegia
diplophonia, dyplophonia
diplopia
dipper curve
direct
  d. current (DC)
  d. laryngoscopy
  d. motor system
  d. selection communication board
directional
  d. microphone
  d. preponderance (DP)
directionality
directivity
disability
  learning d. (LD)
  Slingerland Screening Tests for Identifying Children with Specific Language D.
disassimilation, dissimilation
disassociation, dissociation
discharge
  serosanguineous d.
discoid lupus erythematosus

NOTES

discomfort
> threshold of d. (TD)
> d. threshold

discontinuous neck dissection

discourse

discrimination
> auditory d.
> auditory figure-ground d.
> d. curve
> Goldman-Fristoe-Woodcock Test of Auditory D.
> d. loss
> Picture Sound D.
> Schiefelbush-Lindsey Test of Sound D.
> d. score
> speech d. (SD)
> Testing-Teaching Module of Auditory D. (TTMAD)
> Tests of Nonverbal Auditory D. (TENVAD)
> d. training
> Tree/Bee Test of Auditory D.
> visual d.
> visual figure-ground d.

disease
> acute respiratory d.
> Addison's d.
> Alzheimer's d.
> autoimmune d.
> autoimmune inner ear d.
> Behçet's d.
> Bowen's d.
> calculous d.
> cardiovascular d.
> catarrhal d.
> cat scratch d.
> Chagas' d.
> Chagas-Cruz d.
> collagen-vascular d.
> congenital polycystic d.
> coronary artery d.
> Crohn's d.
> cytomegalic inclusion d.
> dysgenetic polycystic d.
> fibrocystic d.
> Gilchrist's d.
> granulomatous d.
> Graves' d.
> hand-foot-and-mouth d.
> Hansen's d.
> Hashimoto's d.

> HIV-associated salivary gland d. (HIV-SGD)
> Hodgkin's d.
> inflammatory d.
> Jod-Basedow d.
> Kawasaki's d.
> Korsakoff's d.
> locoregional d.
> Lyme d.
> Menetrier's d.
> Ménière's d.
> Mikulicz d.
> mycotic d.
> no evidence of d. (NED)
> nonspecific granulomatous d.
> obstructive airway d.
> occlusive artery d.
> occupational d.
> ototrophic viral d.
> Paget's d.
> parasitic d.
> Parkinson's d.
> Plummer's d.
> polycystic d.
> pulmonary d.
> Rendu-Osler-Weber d.
> rheumatic d.
> Romberg d.
> Sutton's d.
> Thornwaldt's d.
> vertebral-basilar artery d.
> von Recklinghausen's d.
> Winkler's d.

disequilibrium

disfluency (*var. of* dysfluency)

disjunction
> craniofacial d.

disk herniation

diskinesia (*var. of* dyskinesia)

dislocation

disorder
> articulation d.
> attention deficit d. (ADD)
> attention deficit hyperactivity d. (ADHD)
> auditory d.
> auditory processing d.
> behavior d. (BD)
> breathing d.
> central auditory d.
> central language d. (CLD)
> communication d.

communicative d.
conceptual d.
contiguity d.
endocrine d.
endonasal d.
false role d.
fluency d.
functional d.
functional articulation d.
Haws Screening Test for
  Functional Articulation D.
motor d.
olfactory d.
organic articulation d.
perceptual d.
resonance d.
respiratory d.
Screening Test for
  Identifying Central
  Auditory D. (SCAN)
speech d.
voice d.
displaced speech
displacusis
disposable curette
dissection
bilateral neck d.
discontinuous neck d.
elective neck d.
functional neck d. (FND)
hydraulic d.
mediastinal d.
modified neck d. (MND)
neck d.
radical neck d. (RND)
d. snare
suprahyoid neck d.
supraomohyoid neck d.
tongue-jaw-neck d.
two-team d.

dissector
Hurd d.
dissimilation (*var. of*
  disassimilation)
dissociation (*var. of*
  disassociation)
dissociative reaction
dissonance
cognitive d.
distal
distancing
cognitive d.
distinctive
d. feature analysis
d. features
distoclusion
distortion
amplitude d.
figure-ground d.
harmonic d.
intermodulary d.
nonlinear d.
perceptual d.
speech d.
transient d.
waveform d.
distortional bone conduction
distortion-product emission
distoversion
distractibility
distraction
distress
respiratory d.
distribution
complementary d.
contrastive d.
gaussian d.
noncontrastive d.
normal d.
parallel d.

NOTES

disturbance
    Appraisal of Language D.
      (ALD)
    emotional d.
disyllable
diuretic
divergence circuit
diversion
    laryngotracheal d.
diverticulum, pl. **diverticula**
    esophageal d.
    pharyngoesophageal d.
    pulsion d.
    tracheal d.
    traction d.
    Zenker's d.
division
    maxillary d.
    T12 nerve d.
Dix-Hallpike maneuver
dizziness
DL
    difference limen
doctrine
    usage d.
Doerfler-Stewart Test
dominance
    cerebral d.
    lateral d.
dominant language
Donaldson tube
donkey breathing
Doppler
    color-flow D.
    D. effect
    D. phenomenon
    D. shift
Dorello's canal
dorsa (*pl. of* dorsum)
dorsal
    d. lingual artery
dorsalis
    d. pedis-FDMA system
    d. pedis flap
    tabes d.
dorsum, pl. **dorsa**
**Dos Amigos Verbal Language
  Scale**
double
    d. assimilation
    d. consonant
double-cannula tracheostomy tube

**double-lumen suction irrigation
  tube**
double-spoon biopsy forceps
doubling
douloureux
    tic d.
Downes nasal speculum
Down syndrome
doxorubicin
DP
    directional preponderance
drain
    Penrose d.
drainage
    incision and d. (I&D)
    lumbar d.
    retrograde venous d.
    submandibular d.
    d. system
dressing
    hydrocolloid d.
    moustache d.
    Rhinorocket d.
drill
    cobra-head d.
    high-speed d.
    twist d.
drip
    postnasal d.
drooling
droperidol plus fentanyl
drops
    Allergen Ear D.
    Americaine Otic ear d.
    ear d.
    saline d.
    Timoptic ophthalmic d.
drug
    anticonvulsive d.
    non-S-phase specific d.
    nonsteroidal
      antiinflammatory d.
      (NSAID)
    ototoxic d.
    prophylactic d.
    radiosensitizing d.
    S-phase specific d.
drumhead
drum membrane
Drummond
    artery of D.

dry
  d. hoarseness
  d. mouth
DSS
  Developmental Sentence Scoring
DTIC
  dacarbazine
  dimethyltrianzeno-imidazole-
    carboxamide
DTPA
  gadolinium D.
duckbill
  d. voice prosthesis
duct
  Bartholin's d.
  d. cannulation
  cochlear d.
  endolymphatic d.
  frontonasal d.
  intercalated d.
  lacrimal d.
  nasofrontal d.
  nasolacrimal d.
  nasopalatine d.
  parotid d.
  perilymphatic d.
  periotic d.
  pharyngoinfraglottic d.
  Rivinus d.
  saccular d.
  semicircular d.
  Stensen's d.
  submandibular d.
  thoracic d.
  thyroglossal d.
  utricular d.
  utriculosaccular d.
  vestibulo-infraglottic d.
  Wharton's d.
ductule
ductus reuniens

Dunlap cold compression wrap
  system
duodenal
  d. adenoma
  d. ulcer
duodenoscopy
duodenum
duplication
  syllable d.
dura
  d. mater
  d. mater venous sinus
dural venous sinus injury
Dur-A-Sil ear impression material
duration
duty cycle
Dx
  diagnostic therapy
Dyazide
dye
  fluorescein d.
  d. injection
  radio-opaque d.
dynamic
  d. aphasia
  d. computed tomography
  d. posturography
  d. range
dynamometer
dyne
dyplophonia (*var. of* diplophonia)
dysacusis
dysarthria
  ataxic d.
  flaccid d.
  hyperkinetic d.
  parkinsonian d.
  peripheral d.
  somesthetic d.
  spastic d.
dysaudia

NOTES

dyscalculia
dysfluency, disfluency
dysfunction
 brain d. (BD)
 minimal brain d. (MBD)
 neurological d.
dysgenetic polycystic disease
dysgeusia
dysglossia
dysgraphia
dyskeratosis
 benign intraepithelial d.
 d. congenita
 hereditary benign
  intraepithelial d.
 intraepithelial d.
dyskeratotic leukoplakia
dyskinesia, diskinesia
dyslalia
 functional d.
 organic d.
dyslexia
dyslexic
dyslogia
dyslogomathia
dysmathia
dysmetria
 ocular d.
dysnomia
dysosmia
 congenital d.

dysostosis
 mandibulofacial d.
dysphagia
 sideropenic d.
dysphasia
dysphemia
 d. and biochemical theory
dysphonia
 adductor spasmodic d.
 hyperkinetic d.
 spasmodic d.
 spastic d.
 ventricular d.
dysphrasia
dysplasia
 fibrous d.
dysplastic nevus
dyspnea
dyspraxia
dysprosody
dysrhythmia
dystomia
dystonia
dystopia
 orbital d.
dystrophica
 epidermolysis bullosa d.
dystrophy
 muscular d.

E

EA
    educational age
EAC
    external auditory canal
Eagle's syndrome
ear
    artificial e.
    e. canal
    Cargot e.
    cauliflower e.
    e. drops
    external e.
    glue e.
    inner e.
    internal e.
    e. lobule
    middle e.
    e. muffs
    outer e.
    outstanding e.
    protruding e.
    e. speculum
    e. surgery
    swimmer's e.
    telephone e.
    tin e.
    e. training
eardrum
earlobe adipose tissue
earmold
    nonoccluding e.
    open e.
    perimeter e.
    shell e.
    skeleton e.
    standard e.
    vented e.
earmuffs
ear, nose and throat (ENT)
earphone
earplug
earwax
EASIC
    Evaluating Acquired Skills in
      Communication
Eaton-Lambert syndrome
ebonics
EBV
    Epstein-Barr virus
ecchymosis

eccrine spiradenoma
echo
    e. chamber
    cochlear e.
    e. speech
    e. time
echoic operant
echolalia
    delayed e.
    immediate e.
    mitigated e.
    unmitigated e.
echologia
echophasia
echophrasia
ECHO virus
eclecticism
ECoG
    electrocochleography
ecthyma
ectropion
    paralytic e.
eczematoid external otitis
EDA
    electrodermal audiometry
eddying
edema
    angioneurotic e.
    cerebral e.
    facial e.
    inflammatory e.
    labial e.
    laryngeal e.
    Reinke's e.
    retropharyngeal e.
edentulous space
EDRA
    electrodermal response test
      audiometry
edrophonium chloride
educational
    e. age (EA)
    e. audiology
    e. quotient (EQ)
**educationally mentally handicapped
(EMH)**
EEA
    electroencephalic audiometry
EEG
    electroencephalogram

EEM
  Test for Examining Expressive
  Morphology
EEMG
  evoked electromyography
effect
  adaptation e.
  Bernoulli e.
  body baffle e.
  consistency e.
  Doppler e.
  Féré e.
  halo e.
  head shadow e.
  occlusion e.
  off e.
  on e.
  spiral e.
  Wever-Bray e.
effective
  e. amplitude
  e. masking
effector
  e. operation
efferent
  e. motor aphasia
  e. nerve
efficiency
  masking e.
  vocal e.
effort
  e. level
  vocal e.
effusion
  middle ear e.
  otitis media with e. (OME)
EGF
  epidermal growth factor
egocentric
  e. language
  e. speech
eidetic
  e. imagery
eighth
  e. cranial nerve
  e. nerve action potential
    (8AP)
  e. nerve tumor
elastic stain
elasticus
  conus e.
elected mutism
elective neck dissection

electric
  e. current shunting
  e. field
  e. irritability
  e. nerve stimulator
  e. response audiometry
    (ERA)
electrical
  e. artificial larynx
  e. measurement of speech
    production
  e. potential
electroacoustic
electrocautery
electrocochleogram
electrocochleography (ECoG)
electrode
  e. array
  E-Z Clean laparoscopic e.
  LLETZ/LEEP loop e.
  MegaDyne arthroscopic
    hook e.
  Neotrode II neonatal e.
electrodermal
  e. audiometry (EDA)
  e. response test audiometry
    (EDRA)
electrodesiccation
electrodiagnostic study
electroencephalic
  e. audiometry (EEA)
  e. response audiometry
    (ERA)
electroencephalogram (EEG)
electroencephalograph
electroencephalography
electroglottograph
electroglottographic
electrogustometer
electrogustometry
electrolarynx
electrolyte
electromagnetic wave
electromotive force (EMF)
electromyography (EMG)
  evoked e. (EEMG)
electron
  e. beam
  e. microscope
electroneurography
electroneuronography (ENog)
electronic artificial larynx

electronystagmogram
electronystagmography (ENG)
electro-oculography (EOG)
electrophysiology
electrotherapy
elements of performance objective
elevation
    flap e.
    periosteal e.
elevator
    Cottle e.
    Dean periosteal e.
    e. esophagus
    Freer e.
    Freer septal e.
    Joseph periosteal e.
    MacKenty septal e.
eleventh cranial nerve
ELI
    Environmental Language
    Inventory
elicit
elicited imitation
elislon
ellipsis, pl. ellipses
elliptical recess
embed
embedded
    e. clause
    e. sentence
    e. sound
embolism
    air e.
    pulmonary e.
embolization
embolus
    air e.
embryo
embryology
embryonic

EME
    epithelial-myoepithelial
EME carcinoma
emergent
    e. language
EMF
    electromotive force
EMG
    electromyography
EMH
    educationally mentally
    handicapped
eminence
    arcuate e.
    hypobranchial e.
    hypopharyngeal e.
    hypophysial e.
    malar e.
    pyramidal e.
    triangular e.
eminentia
    e. arcuata
    e. triangularis
emissary vein
emission
    distortion-product e.
    nasal e.
    otoacoustic e.
    spontaneous e.
    stimulated e.
emotional disturbance
emphysema
    orbital e.
    subcutaneous e.
empiric
empiricist theory
empyema
encapsulization
encephalitis, pl. encephalitides
    granulomatous amebic e.

NOTES

encephalitis *(continued)*
    mumps e.
    varicella-zoster e.
encephalocele
    tegmental e.
encoder
encoding
    e. communication board
endaural
    e. incision
    e. mastoid incision
    e. retractor
ending
    inflectional e.
endocentric construction
endocrine
    e. disorder
    e. system
endogenous
Endo-grasper
    Babcock E.-g.
    E.-g. by Babcock
endolymph
endolymphatic
    e. duct
    e. hydrops
    e. sac
endolymphatic-subarachnoid shunt
EndoMax endoscopic
  instrumentation
endometriosis
endonasal disorder
endoneurial tube
endoneurium
endo-osseous implant
Endo-Otoprobe
end organ
end-organ of hearing
endoscope
endoscopic
    e. cholangiopancreatography
    e. ethmoidectomy
    e. forceps
    e. sinus surgery
endoscopy
    flexible fiberoptic e.
    nasal e.
    peroral e.
endothelium
    vascular e.
endotracheal
    e. intubation
    e. tube

end-stage nutritional depletion
end-to-side anastomosis
energy
    acoustic e.
    kinetic e.
    potential e.
ENG
    electronystagmography
English
    Black E.
    manual E.
    pidgin Sign E. (PSE)
    Seeing Essential E. (SEE$_1$)
    signed E.
    Signing Exact E. (SEE$_2$)
English/Spanish
    Del Rio Language Screening
      Test, E.
    Toronto Tests of Receptive
      Vocabulary, E.
engraftment
engram
enlargement
    salivary gland e.
ENog
    electroneuronography
enophthalmos
ENT
    ear, nose and throat
enteral feeding
enteric cyst
enterocytopathogenic human orphan
  virus
enterogenous cyst
entity
entity-locative
entrapment
ENTREE disposable CO$_2$
  insufflation needle
enunciate
Environmental
    E. Language Inventory (ELI)
    E. Pre-language Battery
enzyme
    angiotensin-converting e.
      (ACE)
    mitochondrial oxidative e.
    peroxidative e.
EOG
    electro-oculography
eosinophilia
    cytoplasmic e.
eosinophilic granuloma

epaulet flap
epenthesis
epidemiology
epidermal
    e. growth factor (EGF)
    e. growth factor receptor
epidermidis
    Staphylococcus e.
epidermoid
    e. carcinoma
    e. cyst
    e. resection
    e. tumor
epidermolysis bullosa dystrophica
epidural abscess
epigastric artery
epiglottic
    e. reconstruction
    e. tubercle
epiglottis
    absent e.
    bifid e.
epiglottitis
epignathus
epilepsy
    laryngeal e.
    temporal lobe e.
epimyoepithelial island
epimyoepithelium
epinephrine
    racemic e.
epineurial repair
episode
    aphonic e.
epistaxis
epithelia (*pl. of* epithelium)
epithelial
    e. atypia
    e. cicatrization
    e. neoplasm

epithelialization
epithelial-myoepithelial (EME)
epithelial-myoepithelial carcinoma (EME carcinoma)
epithelioid-cell sialadenitis
epithelioid sarcoma
epithelioma
    e. adenoides cysticum
    cystic adenoid e.
epithelium, pl. epithelia
    desquamating e.
    olfactory e.
    respiratory e.
    squamous e.
    supporting cell of
      olfactory e.
epitope
epitympanic air cell
epitympanum
Epstein-Barr virus (EBV)
EQ
    educational quotient
equal loudness contour
equation
    Larmor e.
equidistant
equilibrium
equipment
    American Medical Source
      laparoscopic e.
    Storz e.
    Wolf e.
equivalent
    grammatical e.
    migraine e.
    e. speech reception
      threshold
ERA
    electric response audiometry

NOTES

ERA *(continued)*
    electroencephalic response
      audiometry
    evoked response audiometry
erg
ergometer
ergonovine maleate
ergotamine
Erich arch bar
erosion
error
    articulation e.
    phonemic articulation e.
    phonetic articulation e.
ERV
    expiratory reserve volume
erysipelas
erythema
    e. multiforme
    e. nodosum
erythematosus
    discoid lupus e.
    lupus e.
    systemic lupus e.
erythrocephalgia
erythromycin
erythroplasia
erythroprosopalgia
escape
    e. learning
    nasal e.
    e. reaction
Escherichia coli
esophageal
    e. balloon tamponade
    e. compression
    e. dilatation
    e. diverticulum
    e. hemangioma
    e. hiatus
    e. spasm
    e. speech
    e. sphincter
    e. stricture
    e. varix
    e. voice
    e. web
esophagitis
    herpetic e.
    infectious e.
    peptic e.
esophagocutaneous fistula
esophagogastric hypothermia

esophagoscope
    Jackson e.
    Jesberg e.
esophagoscopy
esophagotrachea
esophagus
    cervical e.
    corkscrew e.
    elevator e.
esorubicin
Essar handle
essential tremor
esthesioneuroblastoma
esthetic
    e. rhinoplasty
    e. septorhinoplasty
Estlander-Abbé flap
17β-estradiol
estriol
estrogen
estrone
ethanol
ethmoid
    anterior e.
    e. bone
    e. bulla
    e. cell
    e. fissure
    e. nerve
    e. ostium
    e. periostitis
    posterior e.
    e. prechamber
    e. punch forceps
    e. sinus
    e. sinusitis
    supraorbital e.
ethmoidal
    e. artery
    e. cell
    e. infundibulum
    e. labyrinth
    e. labyrinth cell
    e. notch
ethmoidalis
    bulla e.
    fovea e.
ethmoidectomy
    anterior e.
    endoscopic e.
    external e.
    internal e.
    intranasal e.

partial e.
total e.
transantral e.
ethmoiditis
chronic e.
ethmoidomaxillary plate
etiology
etymology
eugnathia
eunuchoid voice
eupnea
eustachian
e. tube
e. tube orifice
euthymol
evacuator
SURGILASE ECS.01
smoke e.
evagination
evaluating
E. Acquired Skills in
Communication (EASIC)
E. Communicative
Competence
evaluation
audiological e.
Bekesy Ascending-
Descending Gap E.
(BADGE)
Compton Speech and
Language Screening E.
hearing aid e. (HAE)
Orzeck Aphasia E.
eversion
evoked
e. electromyography (EEMG)
e. response
e. response audiometry
(ERA)
evolutionary phonetics

examination
Boston Diagnostic
Aphasia E.
Denver Articulation
Screening E. (DASE)
neurotologic e.
oral peripheral e.
exanthematous rhinitis
excessive nasality
exchanger
HumidFilter heat and
moisture e.
excimer ultraviolet laser
excision
alar wedge e.
exclamatory sentence
excrescence
executive aphasia
exenteration
exhalation
exocentric construction
exocranial orifice
exogenous
exophoric
e. pronoun
exostosis, pl. exostoses
expansile forceps
expansion
experimental
e. audiology
e. delayed auditory feedback
e. phonetics
expiration
expiratory reserve volume (ERV)
exposure
industrial e.
noise e.
expression
facial e.
expressive
e. aphasia

NOTES

expressive *(continued)*
   e. language
   E. One-Word Picture
    Vocabulary Test
   E. One-Word Picture
    Vocabulary Test-Upper
    Extension
expressive-receptive aphasia
extended
   e. jargon paraphasia
   e. shoulder flap
extension
   Expressive One-Word
    Picture Vocabulary Test-
    Upper E.
   e. semantics
extensor
   e. digitorum longus muscle
   e. hallucis longus muscle
exteriorized
   e. stuttering
external
   e. auditory canal (EAC)
   e. auditory meatus
   e. carotid artery
   e. ear
   e. ethmoidectomy
   e. jugular vein
   e. nasal nerve
   e. otitis
externalization
exteroception
   tactile e.
exteroceptor
extinction

extirpation
extracapsular tissue
extracranial meningioma
extradural abscess
extralaryngeal approach
extraneous
   e. movement
   e. noise
extranodal malignant lymphoma
extraocular muscle
extraosseous chondrosarcoma
extrapolation
extrapyramidal
   e. pathway
   e. system
   e. tract
extravasate
extravasation
extreme hearing loss
extrinsic
   e. muscles of the larynx
   e. muscles of the tongue
extroversion
extrovert
extrude
extrusion
   tube e.
eye
   e. strain
   e. tooth
eyeball
   rectus muscle of e.
eyelid sphincter
E-Z Clean laparoscopic electrode

F
  Fahrenheit
face validity
facial
  f. artery
  f. asymmetry
  f. canal
  f. deformity
  f. edema
  f. excursion measurement
  f. expression
  f. fracture
  f. lipodystrophy
  f. motor nucleus
  f. nerve
  f. nerve branches
  f. nerve crossover
  f. nerve decompression
  f. nerve latency
  f. nerve paralysis
  f. nerve-preserving
    parotidectomy
  f. nerve root
  f. neuralgia
  f. neurinoma
  f. palsy
  f. paralysis
  f. reanimation
  f. recess
  f. spasm
  f. symmetry
  f. synkinesis
  f. traumagram
  f. vein
facies, pl. facies
  adenoid f.
  leonine f.
  mask-like f.
facilitation
  f. of resonance
facioversion
factitive
factor
  B cell differentiating f.
  B cell growth f.
  B cell stimulating f.
  colony-stimulating f. (CSF)
  epidermal growth f. (EGF)
  Green's f.
  growth f.

  hematopoietic growth f.
  hybridoma growth f.
  Klebanoff f.
  lymphocyte activation f.
  macrophage-activating f.
    (MAF)
  macrophage inhibition f.
    (MIF)
  mitogenic f. (MF)
  nerve growth f. (NGF)
  perpetuating f.
  precipitating f.
  predisposing f.
  T cell growth f.
Fahrenheit (F)
failure of fixation suppression
  (FFS)
falciform crest
falciformis
  crista f.
falling curve
fallopian canal
false
  f. fluency
  f. muscle contraction
  f. paracusis
  f. role disorder
  f. threshold
  f. vocal cord
  f. vocal fold
false-negative response
false-positive response
falsetto
  f. voice
falx cerebri
familial
  f. deafness
  f. hearing loss
farad
farcy
fascia, pl. fasciae
  brachial f.
  cervical f.
  interposing f.
  f. lata strip
  f. lata transfer
  parotid f.
  pharyngeal f.
  preparotid f.
  pretracheal f.

fascia *(continued)*
    prevertebral f.
    temporalis f.
    temporoparietal f.
    transversalis f.
    visceral f.
fascial
    f. plane
    f. space
fascicle
    nerve f.
fasciculus, pl. fasciculi
    arcuate f.
fasciitis
    necrotizing f.
    nodular f.
fasciocutaneous
    f. flap
    f. free flap
FAST
    Fein Articulation Screening Test
    Flowers Auditory Screening Test
fastener
    NG strip nasal tube f.
Fastrac lighting
fat
    buccal f.
    orbital f.
    parapharyngeal f.
    periorbital f.
fatigue
    auditory f.
    olfactory f.
    perstimulatory f.
    vocal f.
    voice f.
fauces
    isthmus of f.
FDC
    follicular dendritic cell
FDMA
    first dorsal metatarsal artery
fear
feared word
feature
    f. contrasts process
    distinctive f.'s
    junctural f.
    nondistinctive f.
    phonetic f.
    semantic f.
feedback
    acoustic f.

    afferent f.
    auditory f.
    corrective f.
    delayed auditory f. (DAF)
    experimental delayed
      auditory f.
    haptic f.
    inverse f.
    kinesthetic f.
    negative f.
    f. reduction circuit (FRC)
    simultaneous auditory f.
    tactile f.
feedforward
feeding
    enteral f.
    oral f.
    parenteral f.
    f. tube
feeling-of-knowing
feeling threshold
Fein Articulation Screening Test (FAST)
femoral
    f. artery-saphenous bulb
      region
    f. cutaneous nerve
fenestra, pl. fenestrae
fenestram
    fissula ante f.
    fissula post f.
fenestrated forceps
fenestration
    tracheal f.
fentanyl
    droperidol plus f.
Féré effect
Fer-Will Object Kit
FESS
    functional endoscopic sinus
      surgery
fetal
FEV
    forced expiratory volume
fever
    Malta f.
    Mediterranean f.
    rheumatic f.
    undulant f.
    uveoparotid f.
FFS
    failure of fixation suppression

fiber
nerve f.
f.'s of Rasmussen
secretomotor f.
UltraLine Nd:YAG laser f.
fiberoptic
flexible f.
f. tip
fiberscope
fibrin
fibrocystic disease
fibrocyte
fibroelastic membrane
fibroma
nasopharyngeal f.
ossifying f.
fibromatosis
fibromyoma
fibro-ossification
fibrosarcoma
fibrosis
cystic f.
submucous f.
fibrous
f. band
f. dysplasia
f. histiocytoma
fibular flap
FID
free induction decay
field
f. cancerization
electric f.
free f.
minimum acceptable f.
 (MAF)
minimum audible f. (MAF)
sound f.
fifth cranial nerve
figure-ground
auditory f.-g.

f.-g. distortion
visual f.-g.
figure of speech
fila olfactoria
filiform papilla
filler
film
intraoral occlusal f.
filter
active f.
band-pass f.
high-pass f.
low-pass f.
notch f.
octave-band f.
pass-band f.
power peak f.
third octave f.
tunable notch f.
wave f.
filtered speech
final consonant position
finding
Test of Word f (TWF)
fine motor
fine-needle aspiration
fine-tipped mosquito hemostat
finger agnosia
fingerspelling
finite
f. grammar
fire
St. Anthony's f.
first
f. cranial nerve
f. deciduous molar tooth
f. dorsal metatarsal artery
 (FDMA)
f. premolar tooth
f. sentence
f. word

NOTES

Fisher-Logemann Test of Articulation Competence

fissula
　　f. ante fenestram
　　f. post fenestram

fissura antitragohelicina

fissure
　　ethmoid f.
　　glaserian f.
　　inferior orbital f.
　　infraorbital f.
　　longitudinal cerebral f.
　　orbital f.
　　petrotympanic f.
　　pharyngomaxillary f.
　　pterygomaxillary f.
　　f. of Santorini
　　superior orbital f.
　　tympanomastoid f.

fistula
　　branchial f.
　　chyle f.
　　esophagocutaneous f.
　　intralabyrinthine f.
　　labyrinthine f.
　　oroantral f.
　　orocutaneous f.
　　perilymph f.
　　perilymphatic f.
　　pharyngocutaneous f.
　　preauricular f.
　　salivary f.
　　f. sign
　　thyroglossal f.
　　tracheocutaneous f.
　　tracheoesophageal f.

fistulization

Fitzgerald Key

Five Slate System

fixation
　　intermaxillary f. (IMF)
　　rigid plate f.

fixed
　　f. interval reinforcement
　　　schedule
　　f. ratio reinforcement
　　　schedule

flaccid
　　f. dysarthria
　　f. paralysis

flaccidity

Flagyl

flame
　　manometric f.

flap
　　advancement f.
　　anterior helical rim free f.
　　apron f.
　　arterialized f.
　　axial f.
　　Bakamjian f.
　　bilobed f.
　　bilobed transposition f.
　　bipedicle f.
　　cervical f.
　　cheek f.
　　cheek advancement f.
　　cheek rotation f.
　　composite f.
　　compound f.
　　f. consonant
　　cutaneous f.
　　cutaneous forearm f.
　　deltopectoral f.
　　deltoscapular f.
　　dermal fat free f.
　　dermal fat pedicles f.
　　digastric muscle f.
　　dorsalis pedis f.
　　f. elevation
　　epaulet f.
　　Estlander-Abbé f.
　　extended shoulder f.
　　fasciocutaneous f.
　　fasciocutaneous free f.
　　fibular f.
　　forehead f.
　　free f.
　　fusiform f.
　　glabellar f.
　　glabellar bilobed f.
　　glabellar rotation f.
　　gracilis muscle f.
　　groin f.
　　hemitongue f.
　　horizontal f.
　　iliac crest free f.
　　iliac crest osseous f.
　　iliac crest osteocutaneous f.
　　iliac crest osteomuscular f.
　　internal oblique
　　　osteomuscular f.
　　interpolation f.
　　intraoral f.
　　island f.

jejunal free f.
Karapandzic f.
Koerner f.
lateral trapezius f.
lateral upper arm f.
latissimus dorsi f.
latissimus dorsi muscle f.
latissimus dorsi
  musculocutaneous f.
latissimus dorsi
  myocutaneous f.
latissimus/scapular muscle f.
latissimus/serratus muscle f.
lip switch f.
lower trapezius f.
masseter muscle f.
melolabial f.
mesiolabial bilobed
  transposition f.
midline forehead f.
mucosal f.
muscle-periosteal f.
musculocutaneous f.
myocutaneous f.
myofascial f.
nape of neck f.
nasolabial f.
nasolabial rotation f.
neck f.
f. necrosis
omocervical f.
osteocutaneous f.
osteomyocutaneous f.
parascapular f.
parasitic f.
pectoralis f.
pectoralis major f.
pectoralis major
  myocutaneous f.
pectoralis myofascial f.
pedicle f.

pedicled myocutaneous f.
periosteal f.
pharyngeal f.
platysma myocutaneous f.
radial forearm f.
random f.
rectus abdominis free f.
rectus abdominis muscle f.
regional f.
retroauricular free f.
rhomboid transposition f.
rotation f.
scalp f.
scalping f.
scalp sickle f.
scapular f.
serratus anterior muscle f.
skin f.
temporalis muscle f.
thoracoacromial f.
tongue f.
TRAM f.
    transverse rectus
      abdominis muscle flap
transposition f.
transverse rectus abdominis
  muscle f. (TRAM flap,
  TRAM flap)
trapezius f.
tympanomeatal f.
unipedicled f.
upper trapezius f.
visor f.
flat-bladed nasal speculum
flava
    macula f.
flavus
    Aspergillus f.
flexible
    f. fiberoptic

NOTES

flexible *(continued)*
  f. fiberoptic bronchoscopy
  f. fiberoptic endoscopy
flexion
  f. reflex
FLEXISENSOR sensor
Flexlite
  Zelco F.
flexor
  f. carpi radialis tendon
  f. carpi ulnaris tendon
  f. hallucis longus muscle
flocculonodular lobe
flocculus of cerebellum
floor-of-mouth
  f.-o.-m. closure
  f.-o.-m. lesion
flow
  air f.
  f. loop
  speech sound f.
Flowers
  F. Auditory Screening Test
    (FAST)
  F. Test of Auditory
    Selective Attention
Flowers-Costello Test of Central
  Auditory Abilities
Floxite mirror light
floxuridine (5-FUdR)
fluconazole
fluctuance
fluency
  basal f.
  f. disorder
  false f.
  verbal f.
fluent
  f. aphasia
Fluharty Speech and Language
  Screening Test
fluid
  cerebrospinal f. (CSF)
  oral f.
  periciliary f.
  proteinaceous f.
  serous f.
fluorescein dye
fluoride
  sodium f.
fluoroscopy
5-fluorouracil (5-FU)

flutter
  alar f.
  auditory f.
FM
  frequency modulation
FND
  functional neck dissection
focal keratosis
focus
  tone f.
  vocal f.
  voice tone f.
Fogarty adherent clot catheter
fold
  anterior mallear f.
  aryepiglottic f.
  bowed vocal f.
  false vocal f.
  glossoepiglottic f.
  Herb's f.
  incudal f.
  interossicular f.
  laryngeal f.
  lateral glossoepiglottic f.
  lateral incudal f.
  lateral mallear f.
  mallear f.
  medial incudal f.
  median glossoepiglottic f.
  median thyrohyoid f.
  nasolabial f.
  obturatoria stapedis f.
  pharyngoepiglottic f.
  polypoid degeneration of
    the true f.
  semilunar f.
  stapedial f.
  superior incudal f.
  superior mallear f.
  tensor f.
  thyrohyoid f.
  triangular f.
  true vocal f.
  tympanic f.
  ventricular f.
  vestibular f.
  vocal f.
  white dural f.
foliate papilla
follicular
  f. adenoiditis
  f. carcinoma
  f. cyst

f. dendritic cell (FDC)
f. lymphoid hyperplasia
f. lymphoma
f. tonsillitis
folliculorum
  Demodex f.
fontanele, fontanelle
  posterior f.
footplate
footpound
foramen, pl. **foramina**
  anterior ethmoidal f.
  f. cecum
  f. cecum of tongue
  f. of Huschke
  incisive f.
  f. lacerum
  f. magnum
  mastoid f.
  optic f.
  f. ovale
  posterior ethmoidal f.
  f. rotundum
  f. singulare
  sphenopalatine f.
  f. spinosum
  stylomastoid f.
force
  electromotive f. (EMF)
  gravitational f.
  nerve f.
forced
  f. duction test
  f. expiratory volume (FEV)
  f. vibration
forceps
  Adson f.
  alligator f.
  backbiting f.
  ball f.
  bayonet f.

biopsy f.
bipolar f.
Blakesley f.
Blakesley-Weil upturned
  ethmoid f.
Blakesley-Wilde f.
Brigham 1x2 teeth f.
center-action f.
C. L. Jackson head-
  holding f.
C. L. Jackson pin-bending
  costophrenic f.
cupped f.
Cushing f.
Dennis Browne tonsil f.
double-spoon biopsy f.
endoscopic f.
ethmoid punch f.
expansile f.
fenestrated f.
foreign body f.
Gordon bead f.
iris f.
Jackson approximation f.
Jackson broad staple f.
Jackson button f.
Jackson conventional foreign
  body f.
Jackson cross-action f.
Jackson cylindrical object f.
Jackson double-prong f.
Jackson dull rotation f.
Jackson flexible upper lobe
  bronchus f.
Jackson globular object f.
Jackson papilloma f.
Jackson ring jaw globular
  object f.
Jackson sharp-pointed
  rotation f.
Jansen-Middleton punch f.

NOTES

71

forceps *(continued)*
    Kahler f.
    Kleinert-Kutz bone-cutting f.
    Matthew f.
    optical biopsy f.
    oval f.
    papilloma f.
    Potts-Smith tissue f.
    right-angle f.
    round f.
    Semken f.
    side-biting Stammberger
     punch f.
    side-lip f.
    sister-hook f.
    small cup biopsy f.
    Smith & Nephew Richards
     bipolar f.
    Stammberger punch f.
    S&T lalonde hook f.
    straight f.
    suction f.
    Takahashi f.
    tonsil f.
    Tucker staple f.
    Tucker tack and pin f.
    upbiting f.
    upturned f.
    upward bent f.
    Watson duckbill f.
    Wilde ethmoid f.
fore-glide
forehead flap
forehead-nose position
foreign
    f. accent
    f. body
    f. body forceps
    f. body magnet
    f. body removal
    f. body remover
forked tongue
form
    free f.
    language f.
    f. word
formal
    f. method
    f. universals
formaldehyde (HCHO)
formant
    f. frequency
    singer's f.

formulation
foroblique bronchoscopic telescope
fortis consonant
forward
    f. coarticulation
    f. masking
fossa, pl. **fossae**
    canine f.
    digastric f.
    glenoid f.
    infratemporal f.
    jugular f.
    lacrimal f.
    mandibular f.
    piriform f.
    posterior f.
    f. pterygopalatina
    pterygopalatine f.
    f. of Rosenmueller
    Rosenmueller f.
    saccular f.
    scaphoid f.
    subarcuate f., f. subarcuata
    supratonsillar f.
    temporal f.
    tonsillar f.
    triangular f.
    f. triangularis
    vestibular f.
Fourier analysis
Fourier's law
fourteen-and-six Hertz positive
    spike
fourth cranial nerve
fovea ethmoidalis
fowleri
    Naegleria f.
fracture
    blowout f.
    facial f.
    frontal sinus f.
    Guérin's f.
    hyoid bone f.
    laryngeal cartilage f.
    Le Fort f.
    malar f.
    mandibular f.
    maxillary f.
    midface f.
    nasal f.
    orbital f.
    petrous pyramid f.
    pyramidal f.

temporal bone f.
trimalar f.
tripod f.
zygomatic f.
fragment
Franceschetti's syndrome
Francisella tularensis
Frankfort horizontal line
Frazier incision
FRC
feedback reduction circuit
functional residual capacity
freckle
Hutchinson's f.
free
f. fat graft
f. field
f. field room
f. flap
f. form
f. induction decay (FID)
f. morpheme
f. muscle graft
f. muscle transfer
f. skin graft
f. thyroxin index (FTI)
f. variation
f. vibration
Freer
F. elevator
F. septal elevator
freeze trim
frena (*pl. of* frenum)
French method
frenulum, pl. frenula
f. linguae
lingual f.
frenum, pl. frena, frenums
lingual f.
Frenzel maneuver

frequency
band f.
defined f.
formant f.
fundamental f.
high f. (HF)
infrasonic f.
f. jitter
Larmor f.
low f. (LF)
modal f.
f. modulation (FM)
f. modulation auditory
trainer
natural f.
primary peak f.
range of f.'s
f. range
resonant f.
respiratory f.
f. response
f. response curve
speech f.
f. theory
ultrasonic f.
frequency-place theory
Frey's syndrome
friable vessel
fricative
gliding of f.
groove f.
slit f.
stopping of f.
friction
frictionless
Friedreich's ataxia
frog in the throat
front
f. phoneme
f. routing of signals (FROS)
f. vowel

NOTES

frontal
- f. bone
- f. branch
- f. bulla
- f. furrow
- f. gyri
- f. lisp
- f. lobe
- f. nerve
- f. ostium
- f. plane
- f. process
- f. projection
- f. recess
- f. sinus
- f. sinus fracture
- f. sinusitis
- f. sinus mucocele
- f. sinus septoplasty
- f. sulcus
- f. suture

frontalis muscle paralysis
fronting
- palatal f.

frontoethmoidal cell
frontoethmoidectomy
frontolateral laryngectomy
frontonasal duct
FROS
- front routing of signals

frostbite
frozen section
frustration tolerance
fry
- glottal f.
- vocal f.

FTI
- free thyroxin index

5-FU
- 5-fluorouracil

5-FUdR
- floxuridine

full-denture smile
Fullerton Language Test for Adolescents
full spectrum low cut
full-thickness skin graft
Fu Manchu pattern
fumigatus
- *Aspergillus f.*

function
- affective f.
- articulation-gain f.
- auditory f.
- central auditory f.
- Clinical Evaluation of Language F.'s (CELF)
- differential f.
- language f.
- performance-intensity f.
- referential f.
- semi-autonomous systems concept of brain f.
- speech-motor f.
- visual-motor f.
- f. word

functional
- f. aphonia
- f. articulation disorder
- F. Communication Profile
- f. deafness
- f. disorder
- f. dyslalia
- f. endoscopic sinus surgery (FESS)
- f. hearing loss
- f. neck dissection (FND)
- f. residual capacity (FRC)

functioning
- general intellectual f.

functor
fundamental frequency
fundoplication
- Nissen f.
- f. of Nissen

funduscopy
fungal infection
fungiform papilla
Fungizone
furrow
- frontal f.
- sagittal f.

Furstenberg regimen
furuncle
fusiform flap
fusion
- auditory flutter f.
- binaural f.

Fusobacterium
fuzzy coat

gadolinium
g. DTPA

GAEL
Grammatical Analysis of Elicited Language

gag
g. reflex

gain
acoustic g.
g. control
HAIC g.
HF average full-on g.
peak acoustic g.
g. potentiometer
primary g.
secondary g.

galea

Galen
G. anastomosis
nerve of G.
G. nerve

galeni
ansa g.

Galilean loupe

galli
crista g.

gallstone

galvanic
g. skin resistance
g. skin response (GSR)
g. skin response audiometry (GSRA)

galvanometer

gamma
g. interferon
g. ray

ganciclovir

ganglion, pl. **ganglia, ganglions**
basal ganglia
cervical g.
geniculate g.
Meckel's g.
otic g.
pterygopalatine g.
Scarpa's g.
sphenopalatine g.
spiral g.
submandibular g.
superior cervical g.
vestibular g.

ganglioneuroblastoma
ganglioneuroma
ganglionic blocker
ganglions (*pl. of* ganglion)
gap
air-bone g.
g. detection
nerve g.

garnet
neodymium:yttrium aluminum g. (Nd:YAG)

gastric
g. decompression
g. mucosa
g. outlet obstruction

gastritis
gastroepiploic artery
gastroesophageal reflux
Gastrografin
gastrointestinal
g. adenocarcinoma
g. bleeding
g. carcinoma

gastroplasty
Collis g.

gastroscope
gastroscopy
gastrostomy
g. feeding tube

gaussian
g. curve
g. distribution
g. noise

gauze
Adaptic g.
Telfa g.

gaze
g. nystagmus
g. paresis
g. test

gelatin sponge
Gelfilm
Gelfoam
general
g. anesthesia
g. intellectual functioning
g. linguistics
g. oral inaccuracy
g. phonetics
g. semantics

generalization
    stimulus g.
generalized
    g. intellectual impairment
    g. reinforcer
generative
    g. grammar
    g. semantics
    g. transformational grammar
generator
    artificial sound g.
    noise g.
genetics
geniculate
    g. ganglion
    medial g.
genioglossus muscle
geniohyoid muscle
genitive case
Gentian violet
geriatric
    g. audiology
Gerlach's tonsil
German
    G. measles
    G. method
germinal center
Gerstmann syndrome
gesture language
giant
    g. cell
    g. cell arteritis
    g. cell granuloma
    g. cell tumor
gibberish
Gibson inner ear shunt
Gilchrist's disease
Gilles de la Tourette syndrome
gingiva, pl. **gingivae**
gingivitis
    acute necrotizing
      ulcerative g. (ANUG)
    necrotizing ulcerative g.
    ulcerative g.
glabella
glabellar
    g. bilobed flap
    g. flap
    g. rotation flap
glairy secretion
gland
    g.'s of Bowman
    buccal g.

    buccal mucous g.
    cardiac g.
    labial g.
    labial minor salivary g.
    lacrimal g.
    lingual g.
    minor salivary g.
    mucous g.
    palatal g.
    parathyroid g.
    parotid g.
    pituitary g.
    salivary g.
    serous g.
    sublingual g.
    submandibular g.
    submaxillary g.
    thyroid g.
    von Ebner's g.
glanders
glandular massage
glaserian fissure
glaucoma
glenoid fossa
glide
    vocalic g.
gliding
    g. of fricative
    g. of liquids
global
    g. aphasia
globe
globular collection
globulin
    thyroxine-binding g. (TBG)
globulomaxillary cyst
glomeruli
    olfactory g.
glomus
    g. jugulare
    g. jugulare tumor
    g. tumor
    g. tympanicum tumor
    g. vagale tumor
gloss
glossal
glossectomy
    partial g.
    subtotal g.
    total g.
glossitis
glossoepiglottic
    g. fold

glossograph
glossolalia
glossopalatine
  g. arch
  g. muscle
glossopharyngeal
  g. nerve
  g. neuralgia
  g. press
glossoptosis
glossoschisis
glossotomy
  labiomandibular g.
  median labiomandibular g.
glottal
  g. area
  g. attack
  g. catch
  g. chink
  g. click
  g. cycle
  g. fry
  g. pulse
  g. replacement
  g. stop
  g. stroke
  g. tone
  g. vibration
glottalization
glotte
  coup de g.
glottic
  g. cancer
  g. closure
  g. spasm
  g. squamous cell carcinoma
  g. stenosis
glottic-subglottic squamous cell
  carcinoma
glottidis
  rima g.

glottis
glottograph
gloves
  Biogel surgeons' g.
glucocorticoid
glucosteroid
glue ear
glutamate
glycerol
  G. Test
glycoprotein
glycopyrrolate
gnathic
gnathion
goblet cell
goiter
  multinodular g.
gold
  g. lid load
  25 G. portable CO_2 laser
Goldman-Fristoe Test of
  Articulation
Goldman-Fristoe-Woodcock
  G.-F.-W. Auditory Skills
    Battery
  G.-F.-W. Test of Auditory
    Discrimination
Golgi system
Gomco pump
gondii
  Toxoplasma g.
gonorrhoeae
  Neisseria g.
Goodenough draw-a-man test
Gordon bead forceps
gouge
gout
gracilis
  g. muscle
  g. muscle flap
Gradenigo's syndrome

NOTES

gradient
- g. echo technique
- g. recalled acquisition in the steady state (GRASS)

gradual topic shift

graft
- auricular cartilage g.
- bone g.
- cantilevered bone g.
- cartilage g.
- connective tissue g.
- costal cartilage g.
- cross-facial nerve g.
- free fat g.
- free muscle g.
- free skin g.
- full-thickness skin g.
- muscular g.
- nerve g.
- neuromuscular pedicle g.
- skin g.
- split calvarial g.
- split skin g.
- split-thickness skin g.
- sural nerve g.
- Thiersch g.

grafting
- autogenous g.
- onlay bone g.

grammar
- case g.
- finite g.
- generative g.
- generative transformational g.
- particular g.
- pedagogical g.
- phrase structure g.
- pivot g.
- prescriptive g.
- scientific g.
- traditional g.
- transformational g.
- transformational generative g.
- universal g.

grammatic
- g. closure
- g. method

grammatical
- g. analysis
- G. Analysis of Elicited Language (GAEL)

- g. category
- g. component
- g. equivalent
- g. meaning
- g. morpheme
- g. structure

Gram stain

grand mal

granular cell myeloblastoma

granulation tissue

granule
- mucigen g.
- mucin g.
- serous g.
- sulfur g.
- Zymogen g.

granulocytopenia

granuloma
- cholesterol g.
- contact g.
- eosinophilic g.
- giant cell g.
- histiocytic g.
- lethal midline g.
- midline g.
- necrotizing g.
- paraffin g.
- silicone g.
- traumatic g.

granulomatosis
- Wegener's g.

granulomatous
- g. amebic encephalitis
- g. cheilitis
- g. disease
- g. sialadenitis

graph
- logarithmic g.

grapheme

GRASS
- gradient recalled acquisition in the steady state

gravel voice

grave phoneme

Graves' disease

gravis
- myasthenia g.

gravitational
- g. force
- g. problem

gray (Gy)

great auricular nerve

greater
g. palatine artery
g. petrosal nerve
g. superficial petrosal nerve
g. wing of sphenoid
Green's factor
Grice suture needle
grimace
groin flap
grommet
groove
alar facial g.
g. fricative
intertubercular g.
nasofacial g.
gross
g. motor
g. sound
ground lamella
group
g. audiometer
control g.
grouping
tumor stage g.
growth factor
GSI 16 audiometer
GSR
galvanic skin response
GSRA
galvanic skin response
audiometry

GSW
gunshot wound
guaifenesin
Guérin's fracture
Guillain-Barré syndrome
gullwing incision
Gunning splint
gunshot wound (GSW)
gusher
perilymph g.
gustatory
g. reflex
g. sweating
g. tearing
guttural
g. voice
gutturophonia
Gy
gray
gypoglossal nerve
gyrus, pl. **gyri**
angular g.
frontal gyri
Heschl's gyri
postcentral g.
precentral g.
supramarginal g.
supramarginal angular gyri
temporal g.
transverse temporal gyri

NOTES

habilitation
  audiologic h.
habit
  normal swallowing h.
habitual pitch
habituation
HAE
  hearing aid evaluation
Haemogram blood loss monitor
Haemophilus influenzae
HAIC
  Hearing Aid Industry
    Conference
      HAIC gain
      HAIC output
hair cell
hairy leukoplakia
Hajek incision
halitosis
Haller's cell
Hall-Morris biphase
Hallpike
  H. maneuver
  H. test
hallucination
halo effect
halogen light source
hamartoma
hamulus
handedness
  left-h.
  right-h.
hand-foot-and-mouth disease
hand-held probe
handicapped
  educationally mentally h.
    (EMH)
  multiply h.
  perceptually h.
  trainable mentally h. (TMH)
handle
  Essar h.
  h. of malleus
Hansen
  cells of H.
Hansen's disease
hapaxepy
haplology
haptic
  h. feedback

h. perception
h. system
hard
  h. glottal attack
  h. of hearing
  h. palate
hard-soft palate junction
hard-wire auditory trainer
harelip
harmonic
  h. distortion
harmony process
harshness
harvesting
HAS
  high-amplitude sucking
    technique
Hashimoto's disease
Hasson laparoscopic trocar
Haws Screening Test for
  Functional Articulation Disorder
HCHO
  formaldehyde
HCl
  pseudoephedrine H.
  ranitidine H.
HDP
  high definition power
head
  h. and neck cancer
  h. shadow effect
  h. turn technique
headache
  cluster h.
  muscle contraction h.
  muscle tension h.
  ocular h.
  tension h.
  traction h.
  vascular h.
hearing
  h. aid
  h. aid evaluation (HAE)
  H. Aid Industry Conference
    (HAIC)
  central h.
  h. conservation
  cross h.
  end-organ of h.
  h. impairment

hearing *(continued)*
    h. impairment
    h. impairment degrees
    h. level (HL)
    H. Level scale
    h. loss
    h. protection device (HPD)
    h. protector
    h. science
    h. threshold level (HTL)
    H. Threshold Level scale
Heart pillow infusor
Heerfordt's syndrome
height
    tongue h.
Heimlich
    H. maneuver
    H. tube
helicis
    cauda h.
    spina h.
    sulcus cruris h.
helicotrema
helium neon beam
helix
Helmholtz' place theory
helper
    h. T cell
    h. T-cell count
helper-inducer T cell
helping verb
hemangioendothelioma
hemangioma
    capillary h.
    cavernous h.
    cherry h.
    congenital subglottic h.
    esophageal h.
    hypertrophic h.
    intramuscular h.
    laryngeal h.
    mixed h.
    senile h.
    strawberry h.
    subglottic h.
hemangiopericytoma
    malignant h.
hematoma
    orbital h.
hematopoietic growth factor
hemiface
hemifacial
    h. atrophy

    h. microsomia
    h. spasm
hemiglossectomy
hemilaryngectomy
hemimandible
    h. reconstruction
hemimandibulectomy
hemimaxillectomy
hemiplegia
hemisphere
hemitongue flap
β-hemolytic streptococcus
hemolyticum
    Corynebacterium h.
hemoptysis
    massive h.
hemorrhage
    laryngeal h.
    subarachnoid h.
hemorrhagic
    h. laryngitis
    h. pansinusitis
hemostat
    Dean tonsil h.
    fine-tipped mosquito h.
    Instat collagen absorbable h.
    mosquito h.
hemotympanum
Henle
    spine of H.
heparin
    h. irrigation
hepatitis
    chronic active h.
Herb's fold
hereditary
    h. benign intraepithelial
      dyskeratosis
    h. hemorrhagic telangiectasis
heredity
Hering-Breuer reflex
hernia
    diaphragmatic h.
    hiatal h.
herniation
    disk h.
herpangina
herpes
    h. labialis
    h. simplex
    h. virus
    h. zoster

h. zoster cephalicus
h. zoster ophthalmicus
h. zoster oticus
herpesvirus
herpetic esophagitis
herpetiformis
dermatitis h.
hertz (Hz)
Heschl's gyri
hesitation phenomenon
heterogeneous
h. word
heterograft
heterolalia
heterophemy
heterophile antibody test
heterotopy
hexamethylmelamine
HF
high frequency
HF average full-on gain
HF average SSPL 90
H-flap incision
hiatal hernia
hiatotomy
hiatus
esophageal h.
h. semilunaris
HICROS
high frequency contralateral
routing of signals
hierarchy
response h.
high
h. definition power (HDP)
h. frequency (HF)
h. frequency audiometry
h. frequency contralateral
routing of signals
(HICROS)
h. frequency deafness

h. frequency response
H. Level SISI
h. vowel
high-amplitude sucking technique
(HAS)
Highmore
antrum of H.
high-pass filter
high-speed drill
high-stimulus speech
Hilger facial nerve stimulator
Hilton
laryngeal saccule of H.
hilum
Hinsberg operation
Hiskey-Nebraska Test of Learning
Aptitude
histamine
histiocytic granuloma
histiocytoma
fibrous h.
histiocytosis X
histogram
poststimulus time h.
histopathology
histoplasmosis
historical
h. linguistics
h. phonetics
history (Hx)
HIV
human immunodeficiency virus
HIV-associated salivary gland
disease (HIV-SGD)
HIV-SGD
HIV-associated salivary gland
disease
HL
hearing level
HLA antigen

NOTES

hoarseness
    dry h.
    rough h.
    wet h.
hockey-stick incision
Hodgkin's
    H. disease
    H. lymphoma
holder
    Baumgartner needle h.
    Dale Foley catheter h.
    Dale tracheostomy tube h.
    Lewy laryngoscope h.
    lion jaw bone h.
    speculum h.
    Webster needle h.
Holinger
    H. anterior commissure
      laryngoscope
    H. bronchoscope
Holman-Miller sign
holophrastic utterance
home language
homeostasis
hominis
    Mycoplasma h.
homogenous, homogeneous
    h. word
homograft
    tympanic h.
homograph
homophene
homophone
homorganics
Hood technique
Hopkins rod lens system
horizontal
    h. canal
    h. flap
    h. limb
    h. plane
    h. plate
    h. projection
horizontal-gaze nystagmus
Hormigueros
hormone
    adrenocorticotropic h.
    thyroid h.
    thyroid-stimulating h. (TSH)
    thyrotropin-releasing h.
      (TRH)
horn
    cutaneous h.

Horton's histamine cephalgia
host response
hot potato speech
Hounsfield unit
House-Brackmann classification
Houston Test for Language
    Development
HPD
    hearing protection device
HTL
    hearing threshold level
HTLV
    human T cell lymphotrophic
      virus
Huguier
    canal of H.
Huguier's canal
hum
    sixty-cycle h.
human
    h. immunodeficiency virus
      (HIV)
    h. T cell lymphotrophic
      virus (HTLV)
HumidFilter heat and moisture
    exchanger
humor
    aqueous h.
humoral
    h. control
    h. immunity
hump removal
Hunt's
    H. neuralgia
    H. syndrome
Hurd
    H. dissector
    H. pillar retractor
Hurst bougie
Hürthle cell carcinoma
Huschke
    foramen of H.
huskiness
Hutchinson's freckle
Hx
    history
hyaline cell
hyalinization
hybridoma growth factor
hydraulic dissection
hydrocephalus
    otitic h.

hydrochloride
    meperidine h.
    phenylephrine h.
hydrochlorothiazide
hydrocolloid dressing
hydrops
    cochlear h.
    endolymphatic h.
    labyrinthine h.
    vestibular h.
hydroxyapatite
17-hydroxy corticosteroid
hydroxylase
    arylhydrocarbon h. (AHH)
11β-hydroxysteroid dehydrogenase
hydroxyurea
hygiene
    oral h.
hygroma
    cystic h.
hyoglossus muscle
hyoid
    h. bone
    h. bone fracture
    h. branchial arch
    h. cartilage
hypacusis
hyperactivity
hyperacusis
hyperbaric oxygen
hyperbole
hypercalcemia
hypercapnia
hypercorrect language
hyperesthesia
    h. acoustica
    laryngeal h.
hyperextension
hyperfunction
hyperkeratosis
hyperkinesia

hyperkinesis
hyperkinetic
    h. dysarthria
    h. dysphonia
    h. syndrome
hypernasality
hypernephroma
hyperosmia
hyperplasia
    diffuse h.
    follicular lymphoid h.
    lymphoid h.
    parotid lymph node h.
    polypoid h.
    pseudoepitheliomatous h.
hyperplastic
    h. adenoiditis
    h. laryngitis
    h. mucosa
    h. rhinosinusitis
    h. tonsillitis
hyperrecruitment
hyperrhinolalia
hyperrhinophonia
hypersecretion
hypertension
    benign intracranial h.
    portal h.
hyperthermia
hyperthyroidism
hypertonic
hypertrophic
    h. adenoiditis
    h. hemangioma
    h. laryngitis
    h. rhinitis
    h. scar
    h. tonsillitis
hypertrophy
    pseudomuscular h.
hypervalvular phonation

NOTES

hypervariable region
hyperventilation
    alveolar h.
hypesthesia
hypnosis
hypnotherapy
hypoactivity
hypoacusis
hypobranchial eminence
hypocalcemia
hypofunction
hypogammaglobulinemia
hypoglossal
    h. canal
    h. nerve
hypoglossal-facial transfer
  procedure
hypoglossal-to-facial nerve transfer
hypoglossi
    ansa h.
    nucleus prepositus h.
hypoglottic
hypogonadism
hypokinesia
hypokinesis
hypokinetic
hypologia
hypomagnesemia
hyponasality
hyponasal speech
hypoparathyroidism
hypopharyngeal
    h. eminence
    h. squamous cell carcinoma
    h. stenosis
hypopharynx
hypophonia
hypophrasia

hypophysial, hypophyseal
    h. eminence
hypophysis
hypoplasia
    lingual h.
    mandibular h.
hypoprosody
hypoproteinemia
hyporhinolalia
hyporhinophonia
hyposialorrhea
hyposmia
hypotension
hypotensive agent
hypothalamus
hypothermia
    esophagogastric h.
hypothesis
    network h.
    Whorf's h.
hypothyroidism
    iatrogenic h.
hypotonic
hypotympanum
hypoventilation
    alveolar h.
hypovitaminosis
hypoxemia
hypoxia
hysteria
    conversion h.
hysterical
    h. aphonia
    h. deafness
    h. stuttering
Hy-Tape surgical tape
Hz
    hertz

I
  I. marker
  I. tracing
IAC
  internal auditory canal
IAM
  internal auditory meatus
iambic stress
iatrogenic
  i. cholesteatoma
  i. hearing loss
  i. hypothyroidism
IC
  inspiratory capacity
icons
ictus laryngis
I&D
  incision and drainage
IDC
  interdigitating dendritic cell
ideation
identification
  i. audiometry
  Word Intelligibility by
    Picture I. (WIPI)
ideographs
idioglossia
idiolalia
idiolect
idiopathic
  i. facial paralysis
  i. language retardation
idiosyncratic
  i. meaning
  i. reaction
idiotope
idiotype
IFROS
  ipsilateral frontal routing of
    signals
iliac
  i. crest
  i. crest free flap
  i. crest osseous flap
  i. crest osteocutaneous flap
  i. crest osteomuscular flap
iliocostalis
  i. dorsi muscle
  i. lumborum muscle
ilioinguinal nerve

Illinois
  I. Children's Language
    Assessment Test
  I. Test of Psycholinguistic
    Abilities (ITPA)
illocution
ILSA
  Interpersonal Language Skills
    and Assessment
imagery
  eidetic i.
imaging
  magnetic resonance i. (MRI)
  radionuclide i.
  thallium i.
  time-of-flight i.
  tumor i.
imbalance
  central language i.
  orofacial muscle i.
IMF
  intermaxillary fixation
imitation
  elicited i.
  spontaneous i.
immature
immaturity
  perceptual i.
immediate
  i. echolalia
  i. sentence constituent
immersible video camera
immittance
  i. test
immotile cilia syndrome
immune
  i. adherence
  i. complex
  i. modulation
  i. response
  i. system
immunity
  adaptive i.
  cell-mediated i.
  humoral i.
  innate i.
  tumor-specific
    transplantation i. (TSTI)
immunobiology
immunocompetent site

immunocytochemistry
immunoglobulin
 secretory i.
immunohistochemical study
immunologic memory
immunoperoxidase stain
immunosuppressive agent
immunosurveillance
immunotherapy
impacted cerumen
impaction point
impact sound
impaired
 mentally i. (MI)
impairment
 aphasic phonological i.
 generalized intellectual i.
 hearing i.
 language i.
 mild hearing i.
 moderate hearing i.
 moderately severe hearing i.
 profound hearing i.
 sensory i.
 severe hearing i.
 slight hearing i.
 smell i.
 specific language i.
 speech i.
impar
 plexus thyroideus i.
impedance
 acoustic i.
 i. audiometry
 i. matching
 mechanical i.
 static acoustic i.
impediment
 speech i.
 i. of speech
imperative
 i. mood
 i. sentence
imperception
 auditory i.
impetigo
implant
 endo-osseous i.
 multichannel cochlear i.
 Nucleus multichannel
  cochlear i.
 osteointegrated dental i.
 Silastic i.

single channel cochlear i.
 synthetic i.
implication
 semantic i.
implicit
 i. language
 i. stuttering
implosive
impregnate
impressionistic phonetics
improvement
 speech i.
inaccuracy
 general oral i.
 oral i.
inactivity
 oral i.
inarticulate
incandescence
incident wave
incipient stuttering
incision
 Caldwell-Luc i.
 Conley i.
 cruciate i.
 curvilinear i.
 i. and drainage (I&D)
 endaural i.
 endaural mastoid i.
 Frazier i.
 gullwing i.
 Hajek i.
 H-flap i.
 hockey-stick i.
 inverted-U i.
 Killian i.
 lip-splitting i.
 lower lip-splitting i.
 MacFee i.
 Martin i.
 Pfannenstiel i.
 postauricular i.
 Risdon i.
 Schobinger i.
 sublabial i.
 transmeatal i.
 transmeatal tympanoplasty i.
 U-shaped i.
 Y i.
incisive
 i. canal cyst
 i. foramen
incisor tooth

incisure, incisura
    sagittal i.
incoherence
incompatible behavior
incompetence
    velopharyngeal i.
incomplete cleft palate
incoordination
incudal
    i. fold
    i. ligament
incudostapedial joint
incus
    i. interposition
indefinite vowel
independent clause
index, pl. indices
    articulation i.
    free thyroxin i. (FTI)
    Sciatic Function I.
    Short Increment
      Sensitivity I. (SISI)
    Social Adequacy I. (SAI)
    Speech with Alternating
      Masking I. (SWAMI)
indicative mood
indicator
    thyration i.
indices (*pl. of* index)
indirect
    i. laryngoscopy
    i. motor system
inductance
induction
    i. coil
    i. loop
inductive reactance
inductor
industrial
    i. audiometry

    i. deafness
    i. exposure
inea temporalis
inertia
inertial bond conduction
infantile
    i. aphasia
    i. autism
    i. perseveration
    i. speech
    i. swallowing
infarction
    myocardial i.
infection
    amebic i.
    bacterial i.
    fungal i.
    middle ear i.
    mycobacterial nodal i.
    opportunistic i.
    orbital i.
    periorbital i.
    pneumococcal i.
    respiratory tract i.
    upper respiratory i. (URI)
    upper respiratory tract i.
    viral i.
    wound i.
infectious
    i. esophagitis
    i. mononucleosis
inferior
    i. alveolar nerve
    i. colliculus
    i. concha
    i. constrictor pharyngeal
      muscle
    i. laryngeal artery
    i. laryngeal nerve
    i. maxillary bone
    i. meatal antrostomy

NOTES

inferior *(continued)*
- i. meatus
- i. meatus antrostomy
- i. nasal concha
- i. nasal nerve
- i. oblique muscle
- i. orbital fissure
- i. pharyngeal constrictor
- i. rectus muscle
- i. thyroid artery
- i. thyroid vein
- i. turbinate
- i. turbinated bone
- i. tympanic artery
- i. vestibular nucleus

inferomedial aspect
infiltration
inflammatory
- i. cell
- i. croup
- i. disease
- i. edema
- i. lesion
- i. oncotaxis

inflection
inflectional ending
influenza
- i. A virus

influenzae
- Haemophilus i.

informal method
informed consent
infra-auricular mass
infracture
infraglottic
- i. squamous cell carcinoma

infrahyoid
- i. artery
- i. muscle
- i. strap muscle

infralabyrinthine approach
infraorbital
- i. artery
- i. fissure
- i. nerve

infrasonic
- i. frequency

infraspinatus muscle
infratemporal
- i. fossa
- i. fossa approach
- i. wall

infratrochlear nerve
infraversion
infundibular cell
infundibulotomy
infundibulum
- ethmoidal i.

InfuO.R. drug delivery pump
infusor
- Alton Deal pressure i.
- Heart pillow i.

ingestion
- bismuth i.
- caustic i.

ingrowth
- squamous epithelial i.

INH
- isoniazid

inhalation
- i. method

inhaler
- Nasacort nasal i.

inhibition
- commissural i.

initial
- i. consonant position
- i. lag
- i. masking
- i. string
- i. teaching alphabet

injection
- air i.
- collagen i.
- dye i.
- i. method
- silicone i.
- Teflon i.
- vocal cord i.

injury
- closed head i. (CHI)
- dural venous sinus i.

innate
- i. immunity

innateness theory
inner
- i. ear
- i. ear tack procedure
- i. language
- i. speech

innervation
innominate
- i. artery
- i. line

Innovar

input
    i. signal processor (ISP)
inserter
    ventilation tube i.
insert hearing protection device
insertion
    i. loss
inspiration
inspiratory
    i. capacity (IC)
    i. laryngeal collapse
    i. reserve volume (IRV)
    i. voice
inspissate
Insta-Mold ear protection device
instantaneous power
Insta-Putty silicone ear plug
Instat collagen absorbable
    hemostat
Institute
    American National
        Standards I. (ANSI)
    United States of America
        Standards I. (USASI)
instructional objective
instrument
    Preschool Language
        Assessment I. (PLAI)
instrumental
    i. avoidance act theory
    i. conditioning
instrumentation
    Baxter V. Mueller
        laparoscopic i.
    EndoMax endoscopic i.
insufficiency
    palatal i.
    pulmonary i.
    respiratory i.
    velar i.
    velopharyngeal i.

insufflation
    i. test set
insulin
integration
    binaural i.
    competing messages i.
integrative
    i. language
    i. learning
intelligence
    Pictorial Test of I.
    i. quotient (IQ)
    Test of Nonverbal I.
        (TONI)
    Wechsler Preschool and
        Primary Scale of I.
        (WPPSI)
intelligibility threshold
intelligible
intensity
    sound i.
intentional
    i. marker (I marker)
    i. tremor
intention semantics
interaction
    communicative i.
    social i.
interarytenoid muscle
interaural attenuation
intercalated duct
intercalation
interconsonantal vowel
intercostal
    i. artery
    i. nerve
    i. vessel
intercostalis
    i. externus muscle
    i. internus muscle
interdental lisp

NOTES

interdigitate
interdigitating dendritic cell (IDC)
interference modification
interferon
    gamma i.
interfrontal septum
interiorized stuttering
interjection
interleukin
intermaxillary fixation (IMF)
intermediary nerve
intermediate
    i. nerve
    i. string
    i. structure
intermedius
    nervus i.
intermetatarsal ligament
intermittent
    i. aphonia
    i. reinforcement schedule
intermodal transfer
intermodulary distortion
intermodulation
interna
    nares i.
internal
    i. acoustic meatus
    i. auditory artery
    i. auditory canal (IAC)
    i. auditory meatus (IAM)
    i. auditory vein
    i. carotid artery
    i. diameter
    i. ear
    i. elastic membrane
    i. ethmoidectomy
    i. jugular vein
    i. juncture
    i. maxillary artery
    i. oblique osteomuscular
    flap
    i. pterygoid muscle
    i. spiral sulcus
international
    I. Organization for
      Standardization (ISO)
    I. Phonetic Alphabet (IPA)
    I. Standard Manual
      Alphabet
    I. Test for Aphasia
interneurosensory learning

internum
    ostium i.
internus
    porus acusticus i.
interoceptor
interoral speech aid
interosseous wire
interossicular fold
interpeak latency
**Interpersonal Language Skills and
    Assessment (ILSA)**
interpolation flap
interposing fascia
interposition
    incus i.
    jejunal i.
interrogative sentence
interrupted tracing (I tracing)
interrupter device
intersensory transfer
intersinus septum
intersphenoid septum
interstitial
    i. radiation therapy
    i. word
intertragic notch
intertubercular groove
interverbal acceleration
intervocalic
in-the-ear (ITE)
in-the-ear hearing aid
intimal dehiscence
intonation
    i. contour
intoneme
intra-arterial chemotherapy
intra-aural
    i.-a. muscle reflex
    i.-a. reflex
intracavitary anesthesia
intracellulare
    Mycobacterium i.
    Mycobacterium avium i.
    (MAI)
intracellular keratinization
intracranial tumor
intraepithelial dyskeratosis
intraglandular stone
intralabyrinthine fistula
intramuscular hemangioma
intranasal
    i. ethmoidectomy
    i. polypectomy

intraneural pressure
intraneurosensory learning
intraoperative hearing loss
intraoral
   i. cone
   i. flap
   i. mucosal defect
   i. occlusal film
   i. pressure
intrapleural
   i. pressure
intrapulmonic
intrathoracic
   i. pressure
intratympanic
intravenous (IV)
   i. antibiotic
   i. antibiotic
intraverbal
   i. acceleration
   i. operant
intrinsic
   i. brainstem lesion
   i. muscles of the larynx
   i. muscles of the tongue
introversion
introvert
intrusion
   linguistic i.
intubation
   endotracheal i.
invasion
   perineural i.
   perivascular i.
invasive keratitis
inventory
   Basic Concept I.
   Bowen-Chalfant Receptive
     Language I.
   Carrow Elicited Language I.
     (CELI)

   Clark Picture Phonetic I.
   Environmental Language I.
     (ELI)
   Oral Language Sentence
     Imitation Diagnostic I.
     (OLSID)
   phonetic i.
   Temple University Short
     Syntax I. (TUSSI)
inverse feedback
inverse-square law
inversion
   i. recovery pulse sequence
inverted
   i. ductal papilloma
   i. papilloma
inverted-U incision
inverting papilloma
involuntary
   i. whispering
iodide
iodine
   radioactive i.
iodine-125 seeding
iodine I-123
iodine I-125
iodine I-131
ion
   thiocyanate i.
ionized air
ionizing irradiation
iontophoresis
iothalamate
   meglumine i.
Iowa Pressure Articulation Test
IPA
   International Phonetic Alphabet
Iproplatin

NOTES

ipsilateral
    i. frontal routing of signals (IFROS)
    i. routing of signals (IROS)
IQ
    intelligence quotient
iris forceps
iron-binding protein
iron deficiency
IROS
    ipsilateral routing of signals
irradiation
    ionizing i.
irrigation
    antral i.
    bacitracin i.
    caloric i.
    heparin i.
    sinus i.
    i. system
irritability
    electric i.
    myotatic i.
irritative receptor
IRV
    inspiratory reserve volume
island
    epimyoepithelial i.
    i. flap
    i. frontalis muscle transfer
    myoepithelial cell i.
    skin i.

ISO
    International Organization for Standardization
isochronal
isodense
isodose curve
isogloss
isolated laryngeal candidiasis
isolation
    i. aphasia
isoniazid (INH)
isoperistaltic
isopropyl alcohol
isoproterenol
isotretinoin
ISP
    input signal processor
israelii
    Actinomyces i.
isthmus
    i. of fauces
    i. tympani anticus
    i. tympani posticus
ITE
    in-the-ear
ITPA
    Illinois Test of Psycholinguistic Abilities
IV
    intravenous

J
  joule
Jackson
  J. anterior commissure
    laryngoscope
  J. approximation forceps
  J. broad staple forceps
  J. button forceps
  J. conventional foreign body
    forceps
  J. cross-action forceps
  J. cylindrical object forceps
  J. double-prong forceps
  J. dull rotation forceps
  J. esophagoscope
  J. flexible upper lobe
    bronchus forceps
  J. globular object forceps
  J. laryngoscope
  J. papilloma forceps
  J. ring jaw globular object
    forceps
  J. sharp-pointed rotation
    forceps
  J. steel-stem woven filiform
    bougie
  J. triangular brass dilator
jacksonian seizure
Jackson's syndrome
Jacobson's
  J. nerve
  J. organ
  J. plexus
Jako laryngoscope
James Language Dominance Test
Jannetta retractor
Jansen-Middleton punch forceps
jargon
  j. aphasia
jaw
  lumpy j.
jaw-winking
jejunal
  j. free flap
  j. interposition
Jena method
Jesberg esophagoscope
jitter
  frequency j.

JND
  just noticeable difference
Jod-Basedow disease
Johnson cheek retractor
joint
  cricoarytenoid j.
  cricothyroid j.
  incudostapedial j.
  metatarsal j.
  metatarsophalangeal j.
  temporomandibular j. (TMJ)
**Joliet 3-Minute Speech and
  Language Screen**
Jonah word
Joseph periosteal elevator
joule (J)
J-receptor
jug-handle view
jugular
  j. bulb
  j. chain lymph node
  j. fossa
  j. lymph node
  j. vein
  j. venography
jugulare
  glomus j.
jugum
jumbling
junction
  hard-soft palate j.
  pontomedullary j.
junctional nevus
junctural feature
juncture
  closed j.
  internal j.
  open j.
  phonetics of j.
  plus j.
  terminal j.
just noticeable difference (JND)
juvenile
  j. nasopharyngeal
    angiofibroma
  j. papillomatosis
juxtacapillary receptor

K3-7991 Thornton 360 degree
   arcuate marker
Kahler forceps
Kallmann's syndrome
kanamycin
Kangaroo gastrostomy feeding tube
Kanner's syndrome
kansasii
   Mycobacterium k.
Kaposi's sarcoma
Karapandzic flap
Kartagener's syndrome
Kaufman Assessment Battery for
   Children
Kawasaki's disease
Kay's rhinolaryngeal stroboscope
kc
   kilocycle
K-complex
Keeler-Galilean surgical loupe
Keeler panoramic loupe
keloid
   k. scar
   k. tumor
keratin
keratinization
   intracellular k.
keratinizing squamous cell
   carcinoma
keratitis
   invasive k.
keratoacanthoma
keratoconjunctivitis sicca
keratoma
keratosis, pl. keratoses
   actinic k.
   focal k.
   k. obliterans
   papillary k.
   seborrheic k.
   senile k.
keratotic papilloma
Kerckring
   valves of K.
kernel
   k. sentence
kernicterus
Kernig's sign
Kerrison rongeur
ketoacidosis

ketoconazole
key
   Fitzgerald K.
   k. word method
kidney
Kiesselbach's plexus
killer cell
Killian
   K. frontoethmoidectomy
      procedure
   K. incision
Killian-Lynch suspension
   laryngoscope
kilocycle (kc)
Kindergarten
   K. Auditory Screening Test
   K. Language Screening Test
      (KLST)
kinesics
kinesiology
kinesthesia
kinesthesis
kinesthetic
   k. analysis
   k. cue
   k. feedback
   k. method
   k. motor aphasia
   k. perception
   k. technique
kinetic
   k. analysis
   k. energy
   k. motor aphasia
King operation
kinocilia
Kinzie method
kit
   Fer-Will Object K.
   Set-Op myringotomy k.
Klebanoff factor
Klebsiella rhinoscleromatis
Kleen-Needle system
Kleinert-Kutz bone-cutting forceps
Kleinsasser anterior commissure
   laryngoscope
Klinefelter's syndrome
KLST
   Kindergarten Language
      Screening Test

knife
  Cottle k.
  myringotomy k.
  sickle k.
Knight nasal scissors
knob
  olfactory k.
Koerner flap

Körner's septum
Korsakoff's disease
KTP/532 laser
KTP laser
KTP/YAG laser
kymogram
kymograph

Labbé
vein of L.
labeling
labial
l. assimilation
l. cleft
l. edema
l. gland
l. minor salivary gland
labial-buccal sulcus
labialis
herpes l.
labialization
labiodental
l. area
labioglossolaryngeal paralysis
labiomandibular glossotomy
labioversion
labyrinth
bony l.
ethmoidal l.
membranous l.
osseous l.
otic l.
vestibular l.
labyrinthectomy
labyrinthine
l. fistula
l. hydrops
l. segment
labyrinthitis
circumscribed l.
congenital luetic l.
diffuse serous l.
diffuse suppurative l.
obliterative l.
viral l.
labyrinthotomy
lacerum
foramen l.
Lacri-Lube
lacrimal
l. bone
l. duct
l. fossa
l. gland
l. groove of maxilla
l. probe
l. process
l. sac

lacrimation test
β-lactamase
lactation
lactic dehydrogenase
lactoferrin
lactoperoxidase
LAD
language acquisition device
ladder
abstraction l.
laddergram
Laennec's cirrhosis
LAER
late auditory-evoked response
lag
initial l.
maturational l.
terminal l.
lagophthalmos
LAK
lymphokine-activated killer cell
lallation
lalling
lalopathy
lambdacism
lamella
basal l.
ground l.
lateral l.
lamina
basal l.
l. cribrosa
l. papyracea
reticular l.
spiral l.
laminography
lancet blade
landmark
Landry-Guillain-Barré syndrome
Langerhans' cells
Langhans' cells
Language
L. Assessment, Remediation, and Screening Procedure
L. Modalities Test for Aphasia
L. Processing Test
L. Proficiency Test (LPT)
L. Sampling, Analysis, and Training

language
- l. acquisition device (LAD)
- American Indian Sign L. (AMERIND)
- American Sign L. (Ameslan, ASL)
- automatic l.
- body l.
- l. boundary
- l. center
- Clark-Madison Test of Oral L.
- l. clinician
- Coarticulation Assessment in Meaningful L. (CAML)
- computer l.
- confused l.
- l. content
- delayed l.
- l. development
- deviant l.
- l. difference
- dominant l.
- egocentric l.
- emergent l.
- expressive l.
- l. form
- l. function
- gesture l.
- Grammatical Analysis of Elicited L. (GAEL)
- home l.
- hypercorrect l.
- l. impairment
- implicit l.
- inner l.
- integrative l.
- mathetic function of l.
- native l.
- nonspecific l.
- nonstandard l.
- oral l.
- l. pathologist
- l. pathology
- prelinguistic l.
- Procedures for the Phonological Analysis of Children's L.
- l. processing
- rationalist theory of l.
- receptive l.
- l. sample
- school l.

- Screening Test of Adolescent L.
- Screening Test for Auditory Comprehension of L.
- sign l.
- standard l.
- l. structure
- subcultural l.
- substandard l.
- Test of Adolescent L.
- Tests for Auditory Comprehension of L.-R (TACL-R)
- l. therapist
- true l.
- twin l.
- written l.

Lap Vacu-Irrigator
large-cell lymphoma
Larmor
- L. equation
- L. frequency

laryngeal
- l. abscess
- l. anesthesia
- l. angioleiomyoma
- l. anomaly
- l. artery
- l. atresia
- l. blastomycosis
- l. burn
- l. cancer
- l. carcinoid
- l. carcinoma
- l. cartilage
- l. cartilage fracture
- l. chondroma
- l. cleft
- l. cramp
- l. edema
- l. epilepsy
- l. fold
- l. framework surgery
- l. hemangioma
- l. hemorrhage
- l. hyperesthesia
- l. image biofeedback
- l. mask
- l. motor paralysis
- l. nerve
- l. obstruction
- l. oscillation
- l. paralysis

l. paresthesia
l. perichondritis
l. prominence
l. reflex
l. release
l. respiration
l. saccular cyst
l. saccule of Hilton
l. sensory paralysis
l. spasm
l. stenosis
l. stent
l. stuttering
l. syringe
l. vein
l. ventricle
l. vertigo
l. vestibule
l. web

laryngectomy
anterior partial l.
frontolateral l.
narrow-field l.
near-total l.
subtotal l.
subtotal supraglottic l. (SSL)
total l.
wide-field total l.

larynges (*pl. of* larynx)
laryngis
ictus l.
myasthenia l.
pachyderma l.
ventriculus l.

laryngismus stridulus
laryngitis
acute l.
acute supraglottic l.
chronic l.
hemorrhagic l.
hyperplastic l.

hypertrophic l.
membranous l.
l. sicca
traumatic l.

laryngocele
laryngofissure
laryngograph
laryngography
laryngology
laryngomalacia
laryngopathy
laryngopharyngectomy
partial l. (PLOP)
total l. (TLP)

laryngopharynx
laryngoplasty
sternothyroid muscle flap l.

laryngopyocele
laryngoscope
Benjamin binocular
slimline l.
Benjamin pediatric
operating l.
Dedo l.
Holinger anterior
commissure l.
Jackson l.
Jackson anterior
commissure l.
Jako l.
Killian-Lynch suspension l.
Kleinsasser anterior
commissure l.
Lindholm operating l.
Lynch suspension l.
Weerda distending
operating l.

laryngoscopic view
laryngoscopy
direct l.

NOTES

laryngoscopy *(continued)*
 indirect l.
 laser l.
laryngospasm
laryngostenosis
laryngotracheal
 l. diversion
 l. stenosis
laryngotracheitis
laryngotracheobronchitis
laryngotracheoesophageal cleft
larynx, pl. **larynges**
 artificial l.
 electrical artificial l.
 electronic artificial l.
 extrinsic muscles of the l.
 intrinsic muscles of the l.
 pneumatic artificial l.
laser
 argon l.
 argon tuneable dye l.
 carbon dioxide l.
 CO2 l.
 l. coagulation
 excimer ultraviolet l.
 25 Gold portable CO_2 l.
 KTP l.
 KTP/532 l.
 KTP/YAG l.
 l. laryngoscopy
 Nd:YAG l.
 neodymium:yttrium
  aluminum garnet l.
 PBI MultiLase D copper
  vapor l.
 pulsed yellow dye l.
 Sharplan l.
 SharpLase Nd:YAG l.
 l. surgery
 tuneable dye l.
 UltraPulse surgical l.
late auditory-evoked response
 (LAER)
latency
 acoustic reflex l.
 facial nerve l.
 interpeak l.
lateral
 l. adenoidectomy
 l. canal
 l. canthotomy
 l. cartilage
 l. cricoarytenoid muscle

 l. crus
 dark l.
 l. dominance
 l. glossoepiglottic fold
 l. incisor tooth
 l. incudal fold
 l. lamella
 l. lemniscus
 light l.
 l. lisp
 l. mallear fold
 l. mallear ligament
 l. mastoid bone
 l. neck crease
 l. parotidectomy
 l. pharyngeal space
 l. projection
 l. pterygoid muscle
 l. pterygoid plate
 l. rectus capitis
 l. rectus muscle
 l. sinus
 l. sulcus
 l. thyrohyoid ligament
 l. trapezius flap
 l. trim of the adenoid
 l. upper arm flap
 l. venous sinus (LVS)
 l. vestibular nucleus
 l. wall sphenoid
laterality
 crossed l.
 mixed l.
 l. theory of stuttering
lateralization
 cortical l.
latissimus
 l. dorsi flap
 l. dorsi muscle
 l. dorsi muscle flap
 l. dorsi musculocutaneous
  flap
 l. dorsi myocutaneous flap
latissimus/scapular muscle flap
latissimus/serratus muscle flap
LATS
 long-acting thyroid stimulator
Laurence-Moon-Biedl syndrome
LAV
 lymphadenopathy-associated
  virus
 lymphocyte-associated virus

lavage
    antral l.
law
    Bernoulli l.
    Fourier's l.
    inverse-square l.
    Ohm's l.
    Semon-Rosenbach l.
    Semon's l.
lax
    l. consonant
    l. phoneme
    l. vowel
LD
    learning disability
LDD
    low drain class D
leak
    cerebrospinal fluid l.
    chyle l.
    salivary l.
learning
    l. disability (LD)
    escape l.
    integrative l.
    interneurosensory l.
    intraneurosensory l.
    operant l.
    paired associate l.
    serial list l.
    l. theory
Le Fort fracture
leiomyoma
leiomyosarcoma
leishmaniasis
    mucocutaneous l.
Leksell rongeur
Lell bite block
lemniscus
    lateral l.

length
    mean sentence l. (MSL)
Lengthened-Off-Time (LOT)
lenis
    l. consonant
    l. phoneme
lens
    contact l.
lenticular process
lentigo
    l. maligna melanoma
    l. senilis
leonine facies
leprae
    Mycobacterium l.
leprosy
leptothrica
    mycosis l.
Lermoyez' syndrome
lesion
    cylindromatous l.
    cystic lymphoepithelial
      AIDS-related l.
    floor-of-mouth l.
    inflammatory l.
    intrinsic brainstem l.
    lymphoepithelial l.
    non-neoplastic tumor-like l.
    sessile l.
lesser
    l. palatine artery
    l. petrosal nerve
    l. superficial petrosal nerve
    l. wing of sphenoid
lesson
    trial l.
LET
    linear energy transfer
lethal midline granuloma
leucovorin
leukemia

NOTES

leukokeratosis nicotina palati
leukopenia
leukoplakia
    dyskeratotic l.
    hairy l.
    nondyskeratotic l.
    speckled l.
levamisole
levator
    l. anguli oris muscle
    l. costae muscle
    l. glandulae thyroidea
    muscle
    l. labii superioris alaeque
    nasi muscle
    l. labii superioris muscle
    l. palpebrae superioris
    l. veli palatini
    l. veli palatini muscle
level
    bone conduction l.
    effort l.
    hearing l. (HL)
    hearing threshold l. (HTL)
    loudness l.
    noise interference l. (NIL)
    operant l.
    overall sound l.
    perceived noise l. (PNdB)
    reference zero l.
    saturation sound pressure l.
    (SSPL)
    sensation l. (SL)
    sensorineural acuity l. (SAL)
    sound l.
    sound pressure l. (SPL)
    speech interference l. (SIL)
    threshold hearing l.
    tolerance l.
    uncomfortable l. (UCL)
    uncomfortable loudness l.
    (UCL)
    zero hearing l.
Levy articulating retractor
Lewy laryngoscope holder
lexical
    l. category
    l. meaning
    l. morpheme
    l. word
lexicography
lexicon

LF
    low frequency
lichen planus
lid-loading technique
lidocaine
LIFEMASK infant resuscitator
lift
    palatal l.
ligament
    annular l.
    anterior mallear l.
    anterior suspensory l.
    Berry's l.
    Broyle's l.
    incudal l.
    intermetatarsal l.
    lateral mallear l.
    lateral thyrohyoid l.
    l. of Lockwood
    Lockwood's l.
    mallear l.
    malleosphenomandibular l.
    median thyrohyoid l.
    petroclinoid l.
    posterior incudal l.
    posterior suspensory l.
    sphenomandibular l.
    spiral l.
    superior incudal l.
    superior mallear l.
    suspensory l.
    thyroepiglottic l.
    thyrohyoid l.
    vestibular l.
    vocal l.
ligation
    parotid duct l.
    transesophageal varix l.
light
    cold l.
    cone of l.
    Floxite mirror l.
    l. lateral
    l. voice
    l. vowel
lighting
    Fastrac l.
Lillie-Crow test
limb
    horizontal l.
limen
    difference l. (DL)

l. nasi
temporal difference l. (TDL)
limited
l. range audiometer
l. range speech audiometer
limiter
noise l.
Lindamood Auditory
Conceptualization Test
Lindholm operating laryngoscope
line
Frankfort horizontal l.
innominate l.
middle cranial fossa l.
oblique l.
Ohngren's l.
orbital l.
Reid's base l.
sinus l.
temporal l.
Tycos pressure infusion l.
linear
l. energy transfer (LET)
l. hearing aid
lingua-alveolar
l.-a. area
linguadental (*var. of* linguodental)
linguae
frenulum l.
linguagram
lingual
l. artery
l. frenulum
l. frenum
l. gland
l. hypoplasia
l. lisp
l. nerve
l. paralysis
l. raphe

l. thyroid
l. tonsil
lingualplasty
linguist
linguistic
l. aspect
l. competence
l. component
l. determinism
l. intrusion
l. performance
l. phonetics
l. relativity
l. retention
l. universals
l. variation
linguistics
anthropological l.
applied l.
comparative l.
contrastive l.
general l.
historical l.
theoretical l.
linguodental, linguadental
l. area
linguoversion
lining
oral mucosal l.
linking verb
lion jaw bone holder
lip
bilateral cleft l.
cleft l.
median cleft l.
l. rounding
l. switch flap
unilateral cleft l.
lipase
lipodystrophy
facial l.

NOTES

105

lipoidosis cutis et mucosae
lipoid proteinosis
lipoma
    salivary l.
lipomatosis
liposarcoma
liposuction
lipreading
lip-splitting incision
lipstick sign
liquefaction
liquid
    gliding of l.'s
lisp
    dental l.
    frontal l.
    interdental l.
    lateral l.
    lingual l.
    nasal l.
    occluded l.
    protrusion l.
    strident l.
    substitutional l.
lisping
list
    PBK Word L.'s
    Phonetically Balanced
      Kindergarten Word L.'s
listening
    auditory selective l.
    dichotic l.
    diotic l.
    selective l.
literal paraphasia
lithium
litotes
Little's area
liver spot
live voice audiometry
living
    Communicative Abilities in
      Daily L. (CADL)
LLETZ/LEEP loop electrode
load
    gold lid l.
lobe
    flocculonodular l.
    frontal l.
    occipital l.
    parietal l.
    parotid deep l.
    temporal l.

lobectomy
    thyroid l.
lobular carcinoma
lobule
    ear l.
local
    l. anesthesia
    l. anesthetic
    l. decongestion
localization
    auditory l.
    cerebral l.
localized amnesia
locative
Lockwood
    ligament of L.
    L. ligament
locomotion
locoregional disease
loculation
locution
loft register
logarithm
logarithmic graph
logical
    l. method
    l. operation
logopedics
logopedist
logorrhea
Lombard Test
lomustine (CCNU)
long-acting thyroid stimulator
   (LATS)
longitudinal
    l. cerebral fissure
    l. wave
longitudinalis
    l. inferior muscle
    l. superior muscle
long term memory
longus
    l. capitis muscle
    l. colli muscle
    palmaris l.
Look and Say Articulation Trainer
loop
    flow l.
    induction l.
loquacity
Lorabid
loss
    central hearing l.

conductive hearing l.
discrimination l.
extreme hearing l.
familial hearing l.
functional hearing l.
hearing l.
iatrogenic hearing l.
insertion l.
intraoperative hearing l.
mild hearing l.
moderate hearing l.
moderately severe hearing l.
nerve l.
noise-induced hearing l.
occupational hearing l.
perceptive hearing l.
postlingual profound
  sensorineural hearing l.
profound hearing l.
sensorineural hearing l.
severe hearing l.
slight hearing l.
unilateral hearing l.
weight l.

Lost Cord Club
LOT
Lengthened-Off-Time
Lothrop frontoethmoidectomy
  procedure
loudness
Bekesy comfortable l. (BCL)
l. growth perception
l. level
most comfortable l. (MCL)
l. unit
loudspeaker
loupe
Galilean l.
Keeler-Galilean surgical l.
Keeler panoramic l.
Panoramic l.

low
l. frequency (LF)
l. frequency response
l. vowel
low drain class D (LDD)
lower
l. half headache of Sluder
l. lateral cartilage
l. lip-splitting incision
l. trapezius flap
low-pass filter
LPT
Language Proficiency Test
lubricant
ophthalmic l.
Ludwig's angina
Luer-Lok syringe
Lukens
L. collecting tube
L. trap
lumbar
l. drainage
l. puncture
Lumex
L. recliner
L. Tub Guard Tall
lumpy jaw
lung
l. abscess
l. capacity
l. volume
l. window
lupus
l. erythematosus
l. pernio
l. vulgaris
Luschka's tonsil
LVS
lateral venous sinus
Lyme disease
lymphadenectomy

NOTES

lymphadenitis
   mycobacterial l.
   toxoplasma l.
lymphadenoma
   sebaceous l.
lymphadenopathy
lymphadenopathy-associated virus (LAV)
lymphangiohemangioma
   cavernous l.
lymphangioma
lymphaticovenous anastomosis
lymphedema
lymph node
lymphocele
lymphocyte
   l. activation factor
   B l.
   T l.
lymphocyte-associated virus (LAV)
lymphocytic choriomeningitis
lymphoepithelial
   l. cyst
   l. lesion
   l. proliferation
lymphoepithelioma
   malignant l.
lymphoid hyperplasia

lymphokine
lymphokine-activated killer cell (LAK)
lymphoma
   Burkitt's l.
   diffuse large cell l.
   extranodal malignant l.
   follicular l.
   Hodgkin's l.
   large-cell l.
   non-Hodgkin's l.
lymphomatosa
   struma l.
lymphomatosum
   papillary cystadenoma l.
lymphonodular pharyngitis
lymphoreticular tumor
lymphotoxin
Lynch
   L. frontoethmoidectomy
      procedure
   L. procedure
   L. suspension laryngoscope
lyophilized
   l. dural patch
   l. Transderm Scōp
      transdermal patch
lysozyme

MA
  mental age
MAC
  Minimum Auditory Capabilities
    Test
MacFee incision
MacKenty septal elevator
MacKenzie's syndrome
macrocephaly
macrocheilia, macrochilia
macroglobulinemia
  Wadenstrom's m.
macroglossia
macrognathia
macrophage
  chemotactic factor for m.
    (CFM)
  m. inhibition factor (MIF)
macrophage-activating factor
  (MAF)
macrophonia
macrostomia
macula, pl. maculae
  acoustic m.
  m. cribrosa media
  m. flava
  medial cribrose m.
macular hair cell
MAF
  macrophage-activating factor
  minimum acceptable field
  minimum audible field
Maglite
magnet
  foreign body m.
magnetic
  m. resonance angiography
    (MRA)
  m. resonance imaging
    (MRI)
Magnevist
magnitude
  response m.
magnum
  foramen m.
MAI
  Mycobacterium avium
    intracellulare
main clause

mainstreaming
major histocompatibility complex
  (MHC)
mal
  grand m.
  petit m.
maladaptive response
malar
  m. bone
  m. eminence
  m. fracture
maleate
  ergonovine m.
male-pattern baldness
malformation
  Arnold-Chiari m.
  arteriovenous m. (AVM)
  Bing-Siebenmann m.
  congenital m.
  Michel m.
  Mondini m.
  Mondini-Alexander m.
  Scheibe m.
  vascular m.
malic dehydrogenase
malignant
  m. external otitis
  m. hemangiopericytoma
  m. lymphoepithelioma
  m. melanoma
  m. transformation
malinger
mallear
  m. fold
  m. ligament
mallei
  Pseudomonas m.
malleosphenomandibular
  ligament
malleus
  handle of m.
  m. nipper
malleus-footplate assembly
malleus-stapes assembly
Mallory-Weiss syndrome
malocclusion
  teeth m.
malodor
Maloney bougie
malposition
  teeth m.

Malta fever
mammary artery
management
    airway m.
    contingency m.
mandible
    ascending ramus of the m.
    m. rim
mandibular
    m. arch
    m. cyst
    m. fossa
    m. fracture
    m. hypoplasia
    m. miniplate
    m. nerve
    m. osteotomy
    m. plate
    m. reconstruction
    m. restriction
    m. sieving
    m. swing operation
mandibulectomy
    segmental m.
mandibulofacial dysostosis
mandibulotomy
mand operant
maneuver
    Cairns m.
    Dix-Hallpike m.
    Frenzel m.
    Hallpike m.
    Heimlich m.
    Valsalva m.
maneuverability
manic reaction
manipulation
    digital m.
mannitol
manometric flame
mantle
    blue m.
manual
    m. alphabet
    m. English
    m. method
    m. volume control
manubrium, pl. manubria
MAP
    minimum audible pressure
    Muma Assessment Program
mapping
    auditory brain m.

    brain m.
    cognitive m.
    nerve m.
marginal mandibular nerve
marked falling curve
markedness theory
marker
    I m.
        intentional marker
    intentional m. (I marker)
    K3-7991 Thornton 360
        degree arcuate m.
    sign m.
    tumor m.
Marquette monitor
marsupialization
Martin incision
Masera's septal organ
mask
    laryngeal m.
masker
    tinnitus m.
    tunable tinnitus m.
masking
    backward m.
    central m.
    effective m.
    m. efficiency
    forward m.
    initial m.
    m. level difference
    maximum m.
    peripheral m.
    m. technique
    upward m.
mask-like facies
mass
    infra-auricular m.
massage
    glandular m.
masseter
    m. abscess
    m. muscle
    m. muscle flap
    m. muscle transfer
massive hemoptysis
mast cell
mastication
    m. muscle
masticatory reflex
Mastisol
mastoid
    m. antrum

artificial m.
m. bowl
m. cavity
m. cortex
m. emissary vein
m. foramen
m. notch
m. obliteration operation
m. process
m. tip cell
mastoidectomy
modified radical m.
radical m.
tympanoplasty m.
mastoideum
tegmen m.
mastoiditis
coalescent m.
sclerotic m.
match
perceptual-motor m.
matching
impedance m.
mater
dura m.
material
Dur-A-Sil ear impression m.
mathetic
m. function of language
m. text
matrix, pl. **matrices**
Coloured Progressive
Matrices
m. sentence
matter
particulate m.
Matthew forceps
mattress
Akros m.
D.A.D. m.

m. suture
m. suture otoplasty
maturation
rate of m.
maturational lag
max
PB m.
maxilla, pl. **maxillae**
conchal crest of m.
lacrimal groove of m.
maxillary
m. antrum
m. arch
m. artery
m. bone
m. cyst
m. division
m. fracture
m. ostium
m. restoration
m. sinus
m. sinuscopy
m. sinus cyst
m. sinusitis
m. vein
maxillectomy
maximal
m. contrast
maximum
m. acoustic output
m. amplitude
m. duration of phonation
m. duration of sustained
blowing
m. frequency range
m. masking
m. power output (MPO)
m. stimulation test (MST)
Mayer's view
Mayo stand

NOTES

MBD
>minimal brain dysfunction
>minimal brain dysfunction
> syndrome

McCarthy Scales of Children's Abilities

MCL
>most comfortable loudness

MCLR
>most comfortable loudness range

MCT
>mucociliary transport

mean
>m. length of response (MLR)
>m. length of utterance (MLU)
>m. relational utterance (MRU)
>m. sentence length (MSL)

meaning
>grammatical m.
>idiosyncratic m.
>lexical m.
>transferred m.

measles
>German m.
>three-day m.

measure
>Bilingual Syntax M. (BSM)

measurement
>acoustic immittance m.
>anthropometric m.
>facial excursion m.

meatoplasty

meatus, pl. **meatus**
>acoustic m.
>external auditory m.
>inferior m.
>internal acoustic m.
>internal auditory m. (IAM)
>middle m.
>superior m.

mechanical impedance

mechanism
>balance m.
>speech m.

mechanoreceptor

Meckel's
>M. cave
>M. ganglion

meclizine

Mectra irrigation/aspiration system

media
>acute otitis m. (AOM)
>adhesive otitis m.
>aerotitis m.
>catarrhal otitis m.
>chronic suppurative otitis m.
>macula cribrosa m.
>mucoid otitis m.
>necrotizing otitis m.
>nonsuppurative otitis m.
>otitis m.
>purulent otitis m.
>scala m.
>serous otitis m. (SOM)
>suppurative otitis m.
>tuberculous otitis m.

medial
>m. canthus
>m. cribrose macula
>m. geniculate
>m. incudal fold
>m. nasal concha
>m. pterygoid muscle
>m. pterygoid plate
>m. rectus muscle
>m. turbinated bone
>m. vestibular nucleus

medialization

medialized

median
>m. cleft lip
>m. glossoepiglottic fold
>m. labiomandibular glossotomy
>m. lingual sulcus
>m. longitudinal raphe
>m. sagittal plane
>m. thyrohyoid fold
>m. thyrohyoid ligament

mediastinal dissection

mediastinitis

mediastinoscope
>Carlen's m.
>Tucker m.

mediastinoscopy

mediastinum

mediation
>verbal m.

medicamentosa
>dermatitis m.

Mediterranean fever

medulla
    m. oblongata
medullary artery
MegaDyne
    M. arthroscopic hook
      electrode
    M. electrocautery pencil
megaesophagus
megavoltage
meglumine iothalamate
mel
melaninogenicus
    Bacteroides m.
melanoma
    acral lentiginous m.
    lentigo maligna m.
    malignant m.
    superficial spreading m.
melatonin
Melkersson-Rosenthal syndrome
Melkersson's syndrome
mellitus
    diabetes m.
melody of speech
melolabial flap
melphalan
membranaceous ampulla
membrane
    basement m.
    basilar m.
    cricothyroid m.
    cricovocal m.
    drum m.
    fibroelastic m.
    internal elastic m.
    mucous m.
    otolithic m.
    quadrangular m.
    Reissner's m.
    salpingopalatine m.
    salpingopharyngeal m.

    Shrapnell's m.
    stylomandibular m.
    tectorial m.
    thyrohyoid m.
    tympanic m.
    vestibular m.
membranous
    m. labyrinth
    m. laryngitis
memory
    auditory m.
    immunologic m.
    long term m.
    sequential m.
    short-term m.
    m. span
    visual m.
Menetrier's disease
Ménière's
    M. disease
    M. syndrome
meningeal artery
meningioma
    m. en plaque
    extracranial m.
meningismus
meningitidis
    Neisseria m.
meningitis
    cryptococcal m.
meningocele
meningoencephalocele
meningoencephalomyelitis
    mumps m.
meningovascular syphilis
meniscus, pl. menisci
mental
    m. age (MA)
    m. nerve
    m. retardation

NOTES

mentally
m. impaired (MI)
m. retarded (MR)
meperidine
m. hydrochloride
6-mercaptopurine
Merkel cell carcinoma
Merocel epistaxis packing
Merrill Language Screening Test
mesenchymal
m. neoplasm
m. sarcoma
m. tumor
mesenteric arcade
mesioclusion, mesiocclusion
mesiolabial bilobed transposition flap
mesioversion
mesodermal somite
mesons
pi m.
mesotympanum
messages
competing m.
dichotic m.
diotic m.
Messerklinger technique
metachronous tumor
metacognition
metacommunication
metalinguistic
metal reconstruction plate
metaplasia
cystic oncocytic m.
sebaceous m.
metapragmatic
metastasis, pl. **metastases**
cervical m.
metastasize
metastatic neoplasm
metatarsal
m. bone
m. joint
metatarsophalangeal joint
metathesis
meter
ASSESS peak flow m.
noise exposure m.
sound level m.
vibration m.
volume unit m. (VU meter)
VU m.
volume unit meter

methacholine
methantheline bromide
methimazole
methocarbamol
method
acoupedic m.
acoustic m.
analytic m.
artificial m.
auditory m.
bimodal m.
bisensory m.
Bobath m.
breathing m.
Bruhn m.
chewing m.
combined m.
consonant-injection m.
cross-consonant injection m.
formal m.
French m.
German m.
grammatic m.
informal m.
inhalation m.
injection m.
Jena m.
key word m.
kinesthetic m.
Kinzie m.
logical m.
manual m.
mother m.
Mueller-Walle m.
natural m.
Nitchie m.
numerical cipher m.
odd-even m.
oral-aural m.
plateau m.
plosive-injection m.
Politzer m.
Rochester m.
shadowing m.
simultaneous m.
sniff m.
swallow m.
synthetic m.
systematic m.
threshold shift m.
verbotonal m.

visual m.
Warthin-Starry staining m.
methotrexate (MTX)
methyldopa
methylene blue
methylsulfate
diphemanil m.
methysergide
metoclopramide
metonymy
metrizamide
metronidazole
Metz
M. recruitment test
M. Test for Loudness
Recruitment
MF
mitogenic factor
MHC
major histocompatibility
complex
MI
mentally impaired
Michel malformation
microabscess
microanastomsis
microbar
microcephaly
microcheilia, microchilia
microcystic
m. adnexal carcinoma
microfibrillar collagen
microglossia
micrognathia
microlaryngoscopy
micromanipulator
microspot m.
microneurolysis
microneurorrhaphy
microneurosurgery
microorganism

microphone
directional m.
nondirectional m.
omnidirectional m.
probe tube m.
microphonic
cochlear m.
microphonics
microreconstruction
micros
Peptostreptococcus m.
microscope
electron m.
operating m.
Zeiss m.
Zeiss operating m.
microscopy
binocular m.
microsomia
hemifacial m.
microspot micromanipulator
microstomia
microsurgery
microtia
microtubule
microvascular
m. anastomosis
m. bone transfer
m. decompression (MVD)
m. free flap transfer
microvillar cell
microvilli
microvillus, pl. microvilli
midbrain
middle
m. constrictor pharyngeal
muscle
m. cranial fossa line
m. ear
m. ear effusion
m. ear infection

NOTES

middle *(continued)*
    m. ear muscle reflex
    m. fossa approach
    m. fossa plate
    m. fossa retractor
    m. meatal antrostomy
    m. meatus
    m. pharyngeal constrictor
    m. thyroid vein
    m. turbinate
middle-latency response (MLR)
midface
    m. fracture
    m. trauma
midline
    m. forehead flap
    m. granuloma
mid vowel
MIF
    macrophage inhibition factor
migraine
    basilar artery m.
    m. equivalent
migration
Mikulicz
    M. cell
    M. disease
mild
    m. hearing impairment
    m. hearing loss
Miles Magic Mixture
Millar's asthma
Miller-Yoder Comprehension Test
millisecond (msec)
mimetic muscle
mimic speech
minimal
    m. brain dysfunction
    (MBD)
    m. brain dysfunction
    syndrome (MBD)
    m. contrast
    m. pair
minimum
    m. acceptable field (MAF)
    m. audible field (MAF)
    m. audible pressure (MAP)
Minimum Auditory Capabilities Test (MAC)
MiniOX V pulse oximeter
miniplate
    mandibular m.

Mini speech processor
Minnesota
    M. Preschool Scale
    M. Test for Differential
    Diagnosis of Aphasia
minor salivary gland
misarticulation
misphonia
mispronunciation
misuse
    vocal m.
mitigated echolalia
mitochondrial oxidative enzyme
mitogenic factor (MF)
mitomycin-C
mitoxantrone
mixed
    m. deafness
    m. hemangioma
    m. laterality
    m. nasality
mixture
    Miles Magic M.
    m. theory
MLB
    Monaural Loudness Balance Test
MLR
    mean length of response
    middle-latency response
MLU
    mean length of utterance
MND
    modified neck dissection
mobile septum
mobilization
    stapes m.
Möbius syndrome
modal
    m. auxiliary
    m. frequency
    m. tone
modality
    auditory m.
mode
    transverse
    electromagnetic m. (TEM)
    vocal m.
modeling
moderate
    m. hearing impairment
    m. hearing loss

moderately
  m. severe hearing
    impairment
  m. severe hearing loss
modification
  behavior m.
  interference m.
modified
  m. neck dissection (MND)
  m. radical mastoidectomy
  m. Weber-Fergusson
    procedure
modifier
  biologic response m.
  restrictive m.
modiolus
modulation
  amplitude m. (AM)
  frequency m. (FM)
  immune m.
Modulus CD anesthesia system
mogiphonia
Mohs technique
molar tooth
mold
  Teflon m.
mole
moment
  product m. (r)
momentum
  nuclear angular m.
Mona Lisa smile
monaural
  m. hearing aid
  M. Loudness Balance Test
    (MLB)
Mondini
  M. deformity
  M. malformation
Mondini-Alexander malformation

mongolism
moniliasis
monitor
  ACCUTORR bedside m.
  Colin STBP-780 stress test
    blood pressure m.
  Dinamap Plus
    multiparameter m.
  Haemogram blood loss m.
  Marquette m.
  Multinex ID gas m.
  PASSPORT bedside m.
  Stat-Temp II liquid crystal
    temperature m.
  VISA multi-patient m.
monitored live voice audiometry
monitoring
  m. audiometry
  photoplethysmographic m.
  video m.
monoclonal antibody
monocyte
monocytoid cell
monofascicular nerve
monofilament skin suture
monologue
  collective m.
monomorphic
  m. adenoma
  m. pattern
mononucleosis
  infectious m.
monoplegia
monosyllabic word
Monothermal Caloric Test
monotone
mood
  imperative m.
  indicative m.
  subjunctive m.

NOTES

Morgagni
> sinus of M.
> ventricle of M.

Moro's reflex
morpheaform basal cell carcinoma
morpheme
> bound m.
> free m.
> grammatical m.
> lexical m.
> m. structure rule
> zero m.

morphographemic rule
morphological
morphology
> Test for Examining
> Expressive M. (EEM)

morphophonemic component
morphophonemics
morphotactics
mosquito hemostat
Moss balloon triple-lumen gastrostomy tube
most
> m. comfortable loudness (MCL)
> m. comfortable loudness range (MCLR)

mother method
motility
motion
> brownian m.
> ciliary m.
> range of m. (ROM)
> m. sickness
> simple harmonic m. (SHM)

motivating operation
motivation
motokinesthetics
motor
> m. aphasia
> m. area
> m. disorder
> fine m.
> gross m.
> m. neuron

moustache dressing
mouth
> dry m.
> trench m.

Mouthkote
movement
> ballistic m.
> brownian m.
> compensatory m.
> extraneous m.
> random m.
> smooth-pursuit eye m.
> volition oral m.

MPO
> maximum power output

MR
> mentally retarded

MRA
> magnetic resonance angiography

MRI
> magnetic resonance imaging
> surface-coil MRI

MRU
> mean relational utterance

msec
> millisecond

MSL
> mean sentence length

MST
> maximum stimulation test

MTX
> methotrexate

mucigen granule
mucin granule
mucinous cell adenocarcinoma
mucocele
> frontal sinus m.
> retention m.

mucociliary
> m. drainage pathway
> m. transport (MCT)

mucocutaneous
> m. leishmaniasis
> m. lymph node syndrome

mucoepidermoid
> m. carcinoma
> m. tumor

mucoid
> m. otitis media

mucopolysaccharide
mucopurulent
mucopyelocele
Mucor
mucormycosis
mucosa
> buccal m.
> gastric m.
> hyperplastic m.
> nasal m.

oral m.
respiratory m.
mucosae
lipoidosis cutis et m.
mucosal
m. blood vessel
m. coat
m. cyst
m. flap
m. patch replacement
mucosalize
mucositis
mucous
m. blanket
m. cyst
m. gland
m. membrane
m. otitis
m. plug
m. retention cyst
mucoviscidosis
mucus
nasal m.
olfactory m.
salivary m.
mucus-producing adenopapillary carcinoma
mucus-secreting cell
Mueller-Walle method
muffled voice
muffs
ear m.
multichannel cochlear implant
multiforme
erythema m.
MultiLase D
multilocular
Multinex ID gas monitor
multinodular goiter
multiple
m. endocrine neoplasia

m. myeloma
m. primary
m. sclerosis
multiply handicapped
multisensory
Muma Assessment Program (MAP)
mumps
m. encephalitis
m. meningoencephalomyelitis
muscle
adductor longus m.
adductor magnus m.
alar m.
ansa hypoglossus m.
aryepiglottic m.
arytenoid m.
brachialis m.
brachioradialis m.
buccal m.
buccinator m.
constrictor pharyngeal m.
m. contraction
m. contraction headache
corrugator m.
corrugator supercilia m.
cricoarytenoid m.
cricopharyngeus m.
cricothyroid m.
denervated m.
depressor m.
depressor anguli oris m.
digastric m.
dilator naris m.
extensor digitorum longus m.
extensor hallucis longus m.
extraocular m.
flexor hallucis longus m.
genioglossus m.
geniohyoid m.

NOTES

muscle *(continued)*
glossopalatine m.
gracilis m.
hyoglossus m.
iliocostalis dorsi m.
iliocostalis lumborum m.
inferior constrictor
  pharyngeal m.
inferior oblique m.
inferior rectus m.
infrahyoid m.
infrahyoid strap m.
infraspinatus m.
interarytenoid m.
intercostalis externus m.
intercostalis internus m.
internal pterygoid m.
lateral cricoarytenoid m.
lateral pterygoid m.
lateral rectus m.
latissimus dorsi m.
levator anguli oris m.
levator costae m.
levator glandulae
  thyroidea m.
levator labii superioris m.
levator labii superioris
  alaeque nasi m.
levator veli palatini m.
longitudinalis inferior m.
longitudinalis superior m.
longus capitis m.
longus colli m.
masseter m.
mastication m.
medial pterygoid m.
medial rectus m.
middle constrictor
  pharyngeal m.
mimetic m.
mylohyoid m.
nasal m.
nasalis m.
oblique m.
oblique arytenoid m.
obliquus abdominis
  externus m.
obliquus abdominis
  internus m.
obliquus inferior m.
obliquus superior m.
omohyoid m.
orbicularis m.

orbicularis oculi m.
orbicularis oris m.
palatal m.
palatoglossus m.
palatopharyngeus m.
paravertebral m.
pectoralis major m.
pectoralis minor m.
peroneus tertius m.
pharyngeal constrictor m.
pharyngopalatinus m.
platysma m.
posterior cricoarytenoid m.
procerus m.
pterygoid m.
quadratus labii
  superioris m.
quadratus lumborum m.
rectus abdominis m.
rectus capitis m.
rectus medialis m.
rectus superioris m.
risorius m.
salpingopharyngeus m.
sartoriums m.
scalenus anterior m.
scalenus medius m.
scalenus posterior m.
scalp m.
semimembranous m.
serratus anterior m.
serratus posterior
  inferior m.
serratus posterior
  superior m.
soleus m.
splenius capitis m.
stapedius m.
sternoclavicularis m.
sternocleidomastoid m.
sternocleidomastoideus m.
sternohyoid m.
sternohyoideus m.
sternomastoid m.
sternothyroid m.
sternothyroideus m.
strap m.
styloglossus m.
stylohyoid m.
stylopharyngeus m.
subclavius m.
subcostalis m.

superior constrictor
  pharyngeal m.
suprahyoid m.
temporalis m.
m. tension headache
tensor tympani m.
tensor veli palatini m.
teres major m.
teres minor m.
thyroarytenoid m.
thyroepiglottic m.
thyrohyoid m.
trachealis m.
m. transfer
m. transposition
transverse arytenoid m.
transversus abdominis m.
transversus linguae m.
transversus thoracis m.
trapezius m.
tympanic m.
uvular m.
verticalis linguae m.
vocal m.
vocalis m.
zygomaticus m.
zygomaticus major m.
muscle-periosteal flap
muscular
  m. dystrophy
  m. graft
musculoaponeurotic
musculocutaneous flap
mustard
  nitrogen m.
mutagenic
mutation
  m. voice
mute
  deaf m.

mutism
  elected m.
  voluntary m.
MVD
  microvascular decompression
myasthenia
  m. gravis
  m. laryngis
mycelia
mycobacteria (*pl. of*
  mycobacterium)
mycobacterial
  m. lymphadenitis
  m. nodal infection
Mycobacterium
  M. avium
  M. avium intracellulare
    (MAI)
  M. intracellulare
  M. kansasii
  M. leprae
  M. scrofulaceum
  M. tuberculosis
mycobacterium, pl. **mycobacteria**
  atypical m.
Mycoplasma
  M. hominis
  M. pneumoniae
mycosis leptothrica
Mycostatin
mycotic disease
myectomy
myeloblastoma
  granular cell m.
myeloma
  multiple m.
myiasis
mylohyoid muscle
myoblastoma
myocardial infarction
myocutaneous flap

NOTES

**myoelastic-aerodynamic theory of
    phonation**
myoepithelial
    m. cell island
    m. sialadenitis
myoepithelioma
myofascial
    m. flap
    m. pain dysfunction
    syndrome
myofunctional
    m. therapy
myoma
myoneurotization
myopathic
    m. paralysis

myotatic
    m. irritability
    m. reflex
myotomy
    cricopharyngeal m.
myringitis
    bullous m.
myringoplasty
myringostapediopexy
myringotomy
    m. knife
myrinx
myxedema
myxochondroid stroma

N
   newton
N-180 pulse oximeter
N-200 pulse oximeter
Naegleria fowleri
naeslundii
   Actinomyces n.
nafcillin
naloxone
nape of neck flap
Narcan
narcotic antagonist
naris, pl. **nares**
   anterior n.
   dilator n.
   posterior n.
narrative
   n. speech
narrow
   n. transcription
   n. vowel
narrow-band noise
narrow-field laryngectomy
Nasacort nasal inhaler
nasal
   n. accessory artery
   n. airstream
   n. airway
   n. ala
   n. antrostomy
   n. artery
   n. bone
   n. cavity
   n. conchae
   n. congestion
   n. consonant
   n. coupling
   n. emission
   n. endoscopy
   n. escape
   n. fracture
   n. lisp
   n. mucosa
   n. mucus
   n. muscle
   n. nerve
   n. obstruction
   n. packing
   n. polyp
   n. polyposis

   n. port
   n. process
   n. reconstruction
   n. resistance
   n. resonance
   n. respiration
   n. rustle
   n. septal abscess
   n. septal perforation
   n. septum
   n. snort
   n. speculum
   n. spine
   n. spur
   n. synechia
   n. tamponade
   n. tip
   n. tract
   n. turbulence
   n. twang
   n. uncoupling
   n. valve
   n. vestibule
   n. vestibulitis
   n. vibrissa
nasalance
Nasalcrom
nasalis muscle
nasality
   assimilated n.
   excessive n.
   mixed n.
nasalization
   n. of vowel
nasi
   ala n.
   apex n.
   limen n.
   radix n.
nasion
nasoantral window
nasociliary nerve
nasofacial groove
nasofrontal
   n. duct
   n. orifice
nasogastric tube
nasolabial
   n. flap

nasolabial *(continued)*
   n. fold
   n. rotation flap
nasolacrimal duct
naso-ocular
naso-oral
nasopalatine
   n. duct
   n. duct cyst
   n. nerve
nasopharyngeal
   n. abscess
   n. angiofibroma
   n. bursa
   n. carcinoma
   n. cyst
   n. fibroma
nasopharyngolaryngoscope
nasopharyngoscope
nasopharynx
natal
native
   n. language
nativist theory
natural
   n. frequency
   n. killer cells (NK)
   n. method
   n. phonological process
   n. pitch
NDT
   noise detection threshold
Nd:YAG
   neodymium:yttrium aluminum
   garnet
      Nd:YAG laser
near-total laryngectomy
neck
   n. dissection
   n. flap
   n. of middle turbinate
   n. plucking
   n. torsion
necrosis
   aseptic n.
   flap n.
   rim n.
   wound n.
necrotizing
   n. external otitis
   n. fasciitis
   n. granuloma
   n. otitis media

   n. sialometaplasia
   n. tracheobronchitis
   n. ulcerative gingivitis
NED
   no evidence of disease
needle
   n. aspiration
   n. aspiration cytology
   diathermal n.
   ENTREE disposable CO_2
     insufflation n.
   Grice suture n.
   polypropylene n.
   PROTECT.POINT n.
   Rosen n.
negation
negative
   n. correlation
   n. feedback
   n. reinforcer
   n. response
   n. spike
   n. spike-waves
Neisseria
   N. catarrhalis
   N. gonorrhoeae
   N. meningitidis
neoadjuvant chemotherapy
neodymium:yttrium
   n. aluminum garnet
     (Nd:YAG)
   n. aluminum garnet laser
neoglottic reconstruction
neoglottis
neologism
neomycin sulfate
neonatal
   n. auditory response cradle
neonate
neonatorum
   tetany n.
neoplasia
   multiple endocrine n.
neoplasm
   benign epithelial n.
   benign mesenchymal n.
   epithelial n.
   mesenchymal n.
   metastatic n.
Neo-Synephrine
Neotrode II neonatal electrode
nerve
   abducent n.

acoustic n.
n. action potential
afferent n.
alveolar n.
ampullary n.
n. anastomosis
anterior ethmoid n.
Arnold's n.
auditory n.
auricular n.
auriculotemporal n.
n. cell
cervical sympathetic n.
chorda tympani n.
cochlear n.
n. compression
n. of Cotunnius
cranial n.
n. deafness
deep petrosal n.
efferent n.
eighth cranial n.
eleventh cranial n.
ethmoid n.
n. excitability test (NET)
external nasal n.
facial n.
n. fascicle
femoral cutaneous n.
n. fiber
fifth cranial n.
first cranial n.
n. force
fourth cranial n.
frontal n.
n. of Galen
Galen's n.
n. gap
glossopharyngeal n.
n. graft
great auricular n.

greater petrosal n.
greater superficial
  petrosal n.
n. growth factor (NGF)
gypoglossal n.
hypoglossal n.
ilioinguinal n.
inferior alveolar n.
inferior laryngeal n.
inferior nasal n.
infraorbital n.
infratrochlear n.
intercostal n.
intermediary n.
intermediate n.
Jacobson's n.
laryngeal n.
lesser petrosal n.
lesser superficial petrosal n.
lingual n.
n. loss
mandibular n.
n. mapping
marginal mandibular n.
mental n.
monofascicular n.
nasal n.
nasociliary n.
nasopalatine n.
ninth cranial n.
obturator n.
oculomotor n.
olfactory n.
ophthalmic n.
optic n.
peroneal n.
petrosal n.
phrenic n.
polyfascicular n.
posterior ampullary n.
  (PAN)

NOTES

nerve *(continued)*
    posterior ethmoid n.
    posterior inferior nasal n.
    posterior superior nasal n.
    posterosuperior alveolar n.
    radial n.
    recurrent laryngeal n.
    saccular n.
    second cranial n.
    sensory n.
    seventh cranial n.
    n. sheath
    n. sheath tumor
    sixth cranial n.
    spinal accessory n.
    splayed facial n.
    n. stump
    superficial petrosal n.
    superior laryngeal n. (SLN)
    superior maxillary n.
    superior nasal n.
    supratrochlear n.
    sural n.
    temporal n.
    tenth cranial n.
    terminal n.
    third cranial n.
    thoracic n.
    thoracodorsal n.
    n. transfer
    trigeminal n.
    trochlear n.
    n. trunk
    twelfth cranial n.
    tympanic n.
    upper cervical n.
    vagus n.
    vestibular n.
    vestibulocochlear n.
    vidian n.
    zygomatic frontal n.
    zygomatic temporal n.
nervous
    n. cough
    n. system
nervus intermedius
NET
    nerve excitability test
network hypothesis
neural architecture
neuralgia
    facial n.
    glossopharyngeal n.

    Hunt's n.
    occipital n.
    paratrigeminal n.
    postherpetic n.
    sphenopalatine n.
    trigeminal n.
neurectomy
    cochleovestibular n. (CVN)
    pharyngeal plexus n.
    retrolabyrinthine/retrosigmoid
      vestibular n. (RRVN)
    retrolabyrinthine
      vestibular n. (RVN)
    transcochlear
      cochleovestibular n.
    transcochlear vestibular n.
    transtympanic n.
    tympanic n.
    vestibular n. (VN)
neurilemoma
    acoustic n.
neurinoma, neuroma
    acoustic n.
    facial n.
neuritis
    retrobulbar n.
    vestibular n.
neuroaudiology
neurochronaxic
    n. theory
    n. theory of phonation
neuroepithelium
    olfactory n.
neurofibroma
    paranasopharyngeal n.
    plexiform n.
neurofibromatosis
neurogenic tumor
neurolinguistics
neurologic
neurological dysfunction
neuroma *(var. of* neurinoma)
neuroma
    acoustic n.
neuromotor
neuromuscular
    n. pedicle graft
neuromyography
neuron
    motor n.
neuronal
    n. circuit
    n. survival

neuronitis
 vestibular n.
neuropathy
 diabetic n.
neurophonia
neurophrenia
neuropraxia
neurosis, pl. **neuroses**
neurosyphilis
neurotic
 n. profit
 n. theory of stuttering
neurotization
neurotmesis
neurotologic
 n. examination
neurotologist
neurotransmitter
neurovascular
 n. cross compression
  (NVCC)
neutral
 n. stimulus
 n. vowel
neutralization
 vowel n.
neutroclusion
neutron
 n. beam therapy
 n. therapy
nevus, pl. **nevi**
 blue n.
 dysplastic n.
 junctional n.
 spider n.
 Spitz n.
newton (N)
nexin
NGF
 nerve growth factor
NG strip nasal tube fastener

niche
 round window n.
nicotinic
 n. acid
 n. stomatitis
niger
 Aspergillus n.
nigra
 dermatosis papulosa n.
nihilism
Nikolsky's sign
NIL
 noise interference level
ninth cranial nerve
nipper
 malleus n.
Nissen
 fundoplication of N.
 N. fundoplication
Nitchie method
nitrate
 silver n.
nitrofurantoin
nitrogen mustard
nitroimidazole
NK
 natural killer cells
NMR
 nuclear magnetic resonance
N-nitroso compound
node
 delphian n.
 jugular chain lymph n.
 jugular lymph n.
 lymph n.
 periparotid lymph n.
 postglandular n.
 preglandular n.
 regional lymph n.
 retroparotid lymph n.
 retropharyngeal lymph n.

NOTES

node *(continued)*
    singer's n.'s
    speaker's n.'s
    spinal accessory chin
      lymph n.
    subdigastric lymph n.
    submandibular n.
    submandibular lymph n.
    submental lymph n.
    supraclavicular lymph n.
nodosa
    polyarteritis n.
nodosum
    erythema n.
nodular fasciitis
nodularity
nodule
    polypoid vocal n.
    satellite n.
    screamer's n.
    sessile vocal n.
    singer's n.'s
    speaker's n.'s
    thyroid n.
    vocal n.
    vocal cord n.
no-echo chamber
no evidence of disease (NED)
noise
    ambient n.
    n. analyzer
    background n.
    complex n.
    n. detection threshold
      (NDT)
    n. exposure
    n. exposure meter
    extraneous n.
    gaussian n.
    n. generator
    n. interference level (NIL)
    n. limiter
    narrow-band n.
    pink n.
    n. pollution
    random n.
    saw-tooth n.
    speech n.
    Speech Discrimination
      in N.
    thermal n.
    Tone in N. (TIN)

    white n.
    wide-band n.
noise-induced
    n.-i. damage
    n.-i. deafness
    n.-i. hearing loss
nomenclature
nominal
    n. aphasia
    n. compound
nominative
    n. case
    predicate n.
nonchromaffin paraganglioma
noncontrastive distribution
nondirectional microphone
nondistinctive feature
nondyskeratotic leukoplakia
nonfluency
nonfluent aphasia
non-Hodgkin's lymphoma
nonkernel sentence
nonlinear distortion
non-nasal sound
non-neoplastic tumor-like lesion
nonobtrusive text
nonoccluding earmold
nonoral communication
nonorganic deafness
nonperiodic wave
nonpropositional speech
nonpulsed-current stimulus
nonpurulent
non-reduplicated babbling
nonreinforcement
nonsecreting mucosal cyst
nonsense
    n. syllable
    n. word
nonseptate cavity
nonsonorant
nonspecific
    n. granulomatous disease
    n. language
nonspeech sound
non-S-phase specific drug
nonstandard language
nonsteroidal antiinflammatory drug
    (NSAID)
nonsuppurative
    n. otitis media
nonsyllabic speech sound

nonverbal
n. test
nonvocal
n. communication
norm
cultural n.
normal
n. curve
n. distribution
n. probability curve
n. swallowing habit
n. transition
normative phonetics
norm-referenced test
Northampton charts
Northwestern
N. Syntax Screening Test (NSST)
N. University Children's Perception of Speech Test
nose
n. cleft
nostril
notch
acoustic n.
Carhart n.
ethmoidal n.
n. filter
intertragic n.
mastoid n.
n. of Rivinus
Rivinus' n., rivinian n.
supratragal n.
thyroid n.
tragal n.
notched wave
novel stimulus
noxious stimulus
noy

NSAID
nonsteroidal antiinflammatory drug
NSST
Northwestern Syntax Screening Test
NU Auditory Test Lists 4 and 6
nuclear
n. angular momentum
n. chromation
n. magnetic resonance (NMR)
nucleus, pl. nuclei
n. ambiguous
angular vestibular n.
Bechterew's n.
cochlear n.
Deiters' n.
descending vestibular n.
facial motor n.
n. fasciculus solitarius
inferior vestibular n.
lateral vestibular n.
medial vestibular n.
N. multichannel cochlear implant
periolivary n.
n. prepositus hypoglossi
principal vestibular n.
principle vestibular n.
n. salivatorius superior
Schwalbe's n.
spinal vestibular n.
superior vestibular n.
triangular vestibular n.
ventroposteriorinferior n.
vestibular n.
null
numerical cipher method
nutrition
parenteral n.

NOTES

Nu Voice Club
NVCC
  neurovascular cross compression
nystagmus
  caloric n.
  gaze n.
  horizontal-gaze n.
  optokinetic n.

paroxysmal n.
pharyngolaryngeal n.
positional n.
rotationally-induced n.
spontaneous n.
vestibular n.
nystatin

oat cell carcinoma
object
    o. concept
    o. consistency
    o. permanence
objective
    behavioral o.
    o. case
    o. complement
    elements of performance o.
    instructional o.
    operational o.
    performance o.
    predicate o.
    o. quantity
    o. test
obligatory occurrence
oblique
    o. arytenoid muscle
    o. line
    o. muscle
    o. septum
obliquus
    o. abdominis externus
      muscle
    o. abdominis internus
      muscle
    o. inferior muscle
    o. superior muscle
obliterans
    keratosis o.
obliteration
    total ear o.
obliterative labyrinthitis
oblongata
    medulla o.
obscuration
obscure vowel
observation
obsessive compulsive reaction
obstruction
    airway o.
    gastric outlet o.
    laryngeal o.
    nasal o.
    ostial o.
    upper airway o.
obstructive
    o. airway disease
    o. sialadenitis

obstruent
    o. omission
obtrusive text
obturator
    o. nerve
obturatoria stapedis fold
occipital
    o. artery
    o. bone
    o. lobe
    o. neuralgia
occipitomeatal view
occluded lisp
occlusion
    balloon o.
    dental o.
    o. effect
    transfemoral balloon o.
occlusive artery disease
occuloglandular syndrome
occult
    o. cleft palate
    o. primary
occupational
    o. deafness
    o. disease
    o. hearing loss
Occupational Safety and Health
  Act (OSHA)
occurrence
    obligatory o.
Ochterlony gel diffusion technique
octave
    o. band analyzer
    o. twist
octave-band filter
ocular
    o. dysmetria
    o. dysmetria test
    o. headache
oculomotor
    o. nerve
odd-even method
odontoid process
odontoma
odor
    o. blindness
odynophagia
off effect
off-glide

Ohio Tests of Articulation and Perception of Sounds (OTAPS)
ohm
Ohmeda
    O. continuous vacuum regulator
    O. intermittent suction unit
    O. thoracic suction regulator
Ohm's law
Ohngren's line
ointment
    Aureomycin o.
    bacitracin o.
    chlortetracycline o.
olfaction
olfactometry
olfactoria
    fila o.
olfactory
    o. acuity
    o. bulb
    o. cell
    o. cilium
    o. disorder
    o. epithelium
    o. fatigue
    o. glomeruli
    o. knob
    o. mucus
    o. nerve
    o. neuroepithelium
    o. reflex
    o. tract
    o. vesicle
oligodontia
olivary complex
olivocochlear bundle
OLSID
    Oral Language Sentence Imitation Diagnostic Inventory
OME
    otitis media with effusion
omentum
omission
    obstruent o.
    postvocalic obstruent singleton o.
omnidirectional microphone
Omni laser tip
Omniprep
omocervical flap
omohyoid muscle

OMU
    ostiomeatal unit
oncocyte
oncocytic epithelial cell
oncocytoma
oncocytosis
oncogene
oncotaxis
    inflammatory o.
Ondine's curse
on effect
on-glide
onlay
    o. bone grafting
    o. technique
onodi cell
onomatopoeia
ontogenesis
ontogeny
opacification
open
    o. class
    o. earmold
    o. juncture
    o. quotient
    o. syllable
    o. vowel
    o. word
open-bite
opening
    choanal o.
operant
    autoclitic o.
    o. behavior
    o. behavior theory
    o. conditioning
    echoic o.
    intraverbal o.
    o. learning
    o. level
    mand o.
    o. procedure
    tact o.
    textual o.
    o. therapy
    verbal o.
operating microscope
operation
    Caldwell-Luc o.
    effector o.
    Hinsberg o.
    King o.
    logical o.

mandibular swing o.
mastoid obliteration o.
motivating o.
pull-through o.
sensor o.
operational objective
operculum
operta
rhinolalia o.
ophthalmic
o. lubricant
o. nerve
ophthalmicus
herpes zoster o.
opium smoker's tongue
OPMILAS laser system
opportunistic infection
opposite phase
opposition
o. breathing
o. respiration
OPS
output signal processor
optic
o. canal
o. chiasm
o. foramen
o. nerve
optical biopsy forceps
optimal pitch
optokinetic
o. nystagmus
o. test
OR
orienting reflex
oral
o. antibiotic
o. apraxia
o. atresia
o. cancer
o. cavity

o. communication
o. feeding
o. fluid
o. form recognition
o. hygiene
o. inaccuracy
o. inactivity
o. language
O. Language Sentence
Imitation Diagnostic
Inventory (OLSID)
O. Language Sentence
Imitation Screening Test
(ORSIST)
o. mucosa
o. mucosal lining
o. peripheral examination
o. respiration
o. rinse
o. sphincter
o. stereognosis
oral-aural method
oralism
the oral-nasal acoustic ratio
(TONAR)
orbicularis
o. muscle
o. oculi muscle
o. oris muscle
orbit
orbital
o. abscess
o. apex
o. cellulitis
o. decompression
o. dystopia
o. emphysema
o. fat
o. fissure
o. fracture
o. hematoma

NOTES

133

orbital *(continued)*
    o. infection
    o. line
    o. rim reconstruction
    o. roof
    o. support
orbitomaxillary defect
orbitomaxillectomy
orbitonasal tissue
orchitis
order
    rank o.
organ
    o. of Corti
    end o.
    Jacobson's o.
    Masera's septal o.
    otolith o.
    spiral o.
    vocal o.
    vomeronasal o.
organic
    o. articulation disorder
    o. dyslalia
organism
    pleuropneumonia-like o.
organization
Oriental sore
orientation
orienting reflex (OR)
orifice
    eustachian tube o.
    exocranial o.
    nasofrontal o.
origin
ORL
    otorhinolaryngology
oroantral fistula
orocutaneous fistula
orofacial
    o. muscle imbalance
orolingual
oronasal
oro-ocular
oropharyngeal ulcer
oropharynx
orostoma
ORSIST
    Oral Language Sentence
    Imitation Screening Test
orthodontics
orthographic
orthography

orthopsychiatry
Orticochea scalping technique
Orzeck Aphasia Evaluation
oscillation
    laryngeal o.
oscillator
    bone-conduction o.
oscillopsia
OSHA
    Occupational Safety and Health
    Act
osseous
    o. ampulla
    o. labyrinth
ossicle
    auditory o.
    o. chain
ossicular
    o. chain
    o. chain reconstruction
    o. replacement
ossiculoplasty
    tympanoplasty o.
ossification
ossifying fibroma
osteoblastic sinusitis
osteochondroma
    tracheal o.
osteoclast
osteoclastoma
osteocutaneous flap
osteogenesis
osteogenic sarcoma
osteointegrated dental implant
osteoma, pl. **osteomas, osteomata**
osteomeatal
    o. unit
osteomyelitis
    zygomatic o.
osteomyocutaneous flap
osteophyte
osteoplastica
    tracheopathia o.
osteoplastic frontal sinus procedure
osteoradionecrosis
osteosarcoma
osteosynthesis
osteotome
    Rubin o.
osteotomy
    mandibular o.
osteotympanic bone conduction

ostial obstruction
ostiomeatal unit (OMU)
ostium
>   accessory o.
>   accessory maxillary o.
>   anterior ethmoid o.
>   ethmoid o.
>   frontal o.
>   o. internum
>   maxillary o.
>   posterior ethmoid o.
>   sphenoidal o.

otalgia
>   postherpetic o.
>   referred o.

OTAPS
>   Ohio Tests of Articulation and
>   Perception of Sounds

otic
>   o. capsule
>   o. ganglion
>   o. labyrinth
>   o. vesicle

oticus
>   herpes zoster o.

otitic hydrocephalus
otitis
>   acute diffuse external o.
>   acute localized external o.
>   atelectatic o.
>   chronic diffuse external o.
>   chronic stenosing external o.
>   eczematoid external o.
>   external o.
>   malignant external o.
>   o. media
>   o. media with effusion
>   (OME)
>   mucous o.
>   necrotizing external o.
>   seborrheic external o.

otoacoustic emission
otoconia
otocyst
otolaryngologist
otolaryngology
otolith
>   o. organ

otolithic membrane
otological screening
otology
otomicrosurgical transtemporal
approach
otomycosis
otophyma
otoplasty
>   mattress suture o.

otorhinolaryngology (ORL)
otorrhea
otosclerosis
otoscope
>   Siegle o.

otoscopy
otospongiosis
ototoxic
>   o. drug

ototoxicity
ototrophic viral disease
outer ear
out of phase
output
>   HAIC o.
>   o. limiting potentiometer
>   maximum acoustic o.
>   maximum power o. (MPO)
>   peak o.
>   saturation o.
>   o. signal processor (OPS)

outstanding ear
oval
>   o. curette

NOTES

oval *(continued)*
    o. forceps
    o. window
ovale
    foramen o.
overall sound level
overbite
overeruption
overextension
overflow
overjet
overlapping
overlearning
overload
overmasking
overprojecting nasal tip
overrecruitment
overrestriction
overshoot
    calibration o.

overstatement
overt
    o. response
overtone
Owen's view
oximeter
    ACCUSAT pulse o.
    Datascope pulse o.
    MiniOX V pulse o.
    N-180 pulse o.
    N-200 pulse o.
oxygen
    hyperbaric o.
oxyphilic
    o. adenoma
    o. cytoplasm
ozena
    o. caseosa

pacemaker
pachyderma laryngis
pachyonychia congenita
pack
    Cool Comfort cold p.
packing
    Merocel epistaxis p.
    nasal p.
    p. strip
    Weïmert epistaxis p.
pad
    adenoidal p.
    Passavant's p.
paddle
    cutaneous p.
    skin p.
Paget's disease
pain
    referred p.
    p. syndrome
    p. threshold
pair
    minimal p.
paired
    p. associate learning
    p. syllables
palatal
    p. area
    p. fronting
    p. gland
    p. insufficiency
    p. lift
    p. muscle
    p. paralysis
palate
    bilateral cleft p.
    classification of cleft p.
    cleft p.
    complete cleft p.
    hard p.
    incomplete cleft p.
    occult cleft p.
    partial cleft p.
    primary p.
    p. reconstruction
    p. retractor
    secondary p.
    soft p.
    subtotal cleft p.

    total cleft p.
    unilateral cleft p.
palati
    leukokeratosis nicotina p.
    velum p.
palatine
    p. artery
    p. bone
    p. raphe
    p. tonsil
palatini
    levator veli p.
palatization
palatoglossus muscle
palatogram
palatography
palatomaxillary cleft
palatopharyngeal
palatopharyngeus muscle
palilalia
paliphrasia
palliation
palliative care
pallidum
    Treponema p.
palmaris longus
palpate
palpation
palsy
    Bell's p.
    cerebral p.
    facial p.
PAN
    posterior ampullary nerve
pancreatic carcinoma
pancreatography
pancreozymin
panendoscope
panendoscopy
Panje prosthesis
Panoramic loupe
Panorex
pansinusitis
    hemorrhagic p.
papaverine
papilla, pl. papillae
    filiform p.
    foliate p.
    fungiform p.

papilla *(continued)*
    vallate p.
    p. of Vater
papillary
    p. adenocarcinoma
    p. cyst
    p. cystadenoma
      lymphomatosum
    p. keratosis
papilliferum
    sialadenoma p.
papilloma, pl. papillomas, papillomata
    p. forceps
    inverted p.
    inverted ductal p.
    inverting p.
    keratotic p.
    Schneiderian p.
    tracheal p.
    transitional p.
papillomatosis
    juvenile p.
    recurrent respiratory p.
papillomavirus
papyracea
    lamina p.
paracentesis
paracoccidioidomycosis
paracusis, paracusia
    false p.
    Willis' p.
    p.'s willisiana
paradigm
paradigmatic
    p. response
    p. shift
    p. word
paradoxic turbinate
paraffin granuloma
paraganglioma
    nonchromaffin p.
paraglottic space
parainfluenza virus
paralalia
paralambdacism
paralanguage
paralingual sulcus
paralinguistics
parallel
    p. distribution
    p. talk
paralysis, pl. paralyses

    abductor p.
    adductor p.
    bilateral abductor p.
    bilateral adductor p.
    bilateral laryngeal p.
    bulbar p.
    facial p.
    facial nerve p.
    flaccid p.
    frontalis muscle p.
    idiopathic facial p.
    labioglossolaryngeal p.
    laryngeal p.
    laryngeal motor p.
    laryngeal sensory p.
    lingual p.
    myopathic p.
    palatal p.
    pseudobulbar p.
    pseudolaryngeal p.
    Ramsay Hunt facial p.
    recurrent laryngeal nerve p.
    sensory p.
    spastic p.
    unilateral p.
    unilateral abductor p.
    unilateral adductor p.
    vocal cord p.
    vocal fold p.
paralytic
    p. agent
    p. ectropion
paramedical
parameter
paranasal sinus
paranasopharyngeal neurofibroma
paranoia
paranoid reaction
parapharyngeal
    p. fat
    p. space
    p. space abscess
paraphasia
    extended jargon p.
    literal p.
paraphrasia
    verbal p.
paraplegia
pararhotacism
parascapular flap
parasigmatism

parasitic
   p. disease
   p. flap
parasympathetic pathway
parasympatholytic
parasympathomimetic
parasymphyseal region
paratenon
parathyroid
   p. adenoma
   p. gland
paratope
paratrigeminal neuralgia
paravertebral muscle
parenchyma
parenteral
   p. feeding
   p. nutrition
paresis
   gaze p.
paresthesia
   laryngeal p.
parietal
   p. bone
   p. lobe
Parinaud's syndrome
park-bench position
parkinsonian dysarthria
parkinsonism
Parkinson's disease
parosmia
parotid
   p. capsule
   p. carcinoma
   p. collector
   p. deep lobe
   p. duct
   p. duct ligation
   p. duct transposition

   p. fascia
   p. gland
   p. gland abscess
   p. lymph node hyperplasia
   p. resection
parotidectomy
   facial nerve-preserving p.
   lateral p.
   superficial p.
parotin
parotitis
   acute suppurative p.
   suppurative p.
paroxysmal
   p. nystagmus
   p. positional vertigo
Parsons Language Sample
partial
   p. cleft palate
   p. ethmoidectomy
   p. glossectomy
   p. laryngopharyngectomy
     (PLOP)
   p. ossicular prosthesis
   p. ossicular replacement
     prosthesis
   p. recruitment
   p. reinforcement
   p. tone
   upper p.
particle
   p. velocity
particular grammar
particulate matter
partition
   cochlear p.
parts of speech
PAS
   periodic acid-Schiff

NOTES

PASES
  Performance Assessment of
  Syntax Elicited and
  Spontaneous
Passavant's
  P. bar
  P. cushion
  P. pad
pass-band filter
passive
  p. bilingualism
  p. voice
PASSPORT bedside monitor
PAT
  Photo Articulation Test
patch
  lyophilized dural p.
  lyophilized Transderm Scōp
  transdermal p.
patency
Paterson-Kelly syndrome
pathogen
pathogenesis
pathologic
pathologist
  language p.
  speech p.
  speech and language p.
  voice p.
pathology
  language p.
  speech p.
  speech and language p.
pathophysiology
pathway
  auditory p.
  extrapyramidal p.
  mucociliary drainage p.
  parasympathetic p.
  supranuclear p.
  vestibular p.
pathy
  arachidonic acid p.
pattern
  acoustic reflex p.
  auditory p.
  Fu Manchu p.
  monomorphic p.
  pressure p.
  stress p.
  stuttering p.
  variegated p.

**Patterned Elicitation Syntax
  Screening Test (PESST)**
patterning
Paul-Bunnell test
PB
  phonetically balanced
  PB max
  PB word
**PBI MultiLase D copper vapor
  laser**
PBK Word Lists
PE
  pharyngoesophageal
Peabody Picture Vocabulary Test
peak
  p. acoustic gain
  p. clipping
  p. output
pearl
  cholesteatoma p.
**Pearson product-moment coefficient
  of correlation**
pectoralis
  p. flap
  p. major flap
  p. major muscle
  p. major myocutaneous flap
  p. minor muscle
  p. myofascial flap
pedagogical grammar
pediatric
  p. audiology
**Pediatric Speech Intelligibility Test
  (PSI)**
pedicle
  circumflex scapular p.
  p. flap
  transverse cervical p.
  vascular p.
pedicled
  p. colon transfer
  p. enteric donor site
  p. jejunal reconstruction
  p. myocutaneous flap
  p. polyp
pedolalia
pedunculated polyp
**Pegasus Airwave pressure relief
  system**
pellagra
pemphigoid
  bullous p.

pemphigus
>p. vegetans
>p. vulgaris

penalty, frustration, anxiety, guilt, and hostility (PFAGH)

pencil
>MegaDyne electrocautery p.

penicillamine
penicillin
Penrose drain
pentamidine
pentobarbital
peptic
>p. esophagitis
>p. ulcer

Peptostreptococcus
>*P. micros*

perceived noise level (PNdB)
percentage
percentile
>p. rank

perception
>auditory p.
>central auditory p.
>cross-modality p.
>haptic p.
>kinesthetic p.
>loudness growth p.
>Screening Test for Auditory P.
>speech p.
>supramodal p.
>tactile p.
>tactile kinesthetic p.
>visual p.

perceptive hearing loss
perceptual
>p. analysis
>p. consistency
>p. disorder
>p. distortion

>p. immaturity
>p. retardation

perceptually handicapped
perceptual-motor
>p.-m. match

perforation
>nasal septal p.
>septal p.

performance
>P. Assessment of Syntax Elicited and Spontaneous (PASES)
>linguistic p.
>p. objective
>p. test
>Test of Articulation P.-Diagnostic (TAP-D)
>Test of Articulation P.-Screen (TAP-S)

performance-intensity
>p.-i. function
>p.-i. function test

performative
>p. pragmatic structure

periadenitis aphthae
perichondritis
>arytenoid p.
>laryngeal p.

perichondrium
periciliary fluid
pericranium
perilymph
>p. fistula
>p. gusher
>p. protein

perilymphatic
>p. duct
>p. fistula

perimeter earmold
perinatal
perineural invasion

NOTES

141

perineurium
period
  concrete operations p.
  decay p.
  developmental p.
  preoperational thought p.
  refractory p.
  sensorimotor intelligence p.
periodic
  p. acid-Schiff (PAS)
  p. wave
periodicity
periolivary nucleus
perioral
periorbita
periorbital
  p. cellulitis
  p. fat
  p. infection
periosteal
  p. cyst
  p. elevation
  p. flap
periosteum
periostitis
  ethmoid p.
periotic duct
periparotid lymph node
peripharyngeal space
peripheral
  p. apnea
  p. dysarthria
  p. lymphoid tissue
  p. masking
  p. nervous system (PNS)
periphery
perisinus abscess
peristalsis
  residual dyskinetic p.
peritenon
peritonsillar
  p. abscess
  p. cellulitis
perivascular invasion
perlocution
permanence
  object p.
permanent
  p. threshold shift (PTS)
  p. tooth
permeation
per mucosal needle aspiration
permutation

pernio
  lupus p.
peroneal
  p. nerve
peroneus tertius muscle
peroral endoscopy
peroxidase
  salivary p.
peroxidative enzyme
perpendicular
  p. anterior wall
  p. plane
  p. plate
perpetuating factor
perseveration
  infantile p.
  p. theory
personification
Personna Plus disposable Teflon
  scalpel
perstimulatory fatigue
perturbation
pertussis
  Bordetella *p.*
pes anserinus
PESST
  Patterned Elicitation Syntax
  Screening Test
petiole
petit mal
petroclinoid ligament
petroclival
  p. area
petromastoid
petrosal
  p. artery
  p. nerve
  p. ridge
  p. sulcus
petrositis
petrotympanic fissure
petrous
  p. apex tumor
  p. apicectomy
  p. pyramid
  p. pyramid fracture
  p. ridge
PFAGH
  penalty, frustration, anxiety,
  guilt, and hostility
Pfannenstiel incision
PGSR
  psychogalvanic skin response

PGSRA
    psychogalvanic skin response
    audiometry
pH
    salivary p.
phantom speech
pharyngeal
    p. artery
    p. bursa
    p. constrictor muscle
    p. fascia
    p. flap
    p. plexus neurectomy
    p. raphe
    p. recess
    p. reflex
    p. speech
    p. tonsil
    p. vein
pharyngectomy
pharynges (*pl. of* pharynx)
pharyngitis
    lymphonodular p.
pharyngocutaneous fistula
pharyngoepiglottic fold
pharyngoesophageal (PE)
    p. diverticulum
    p. reconstruction
pharyngoinfraglottic duct
pharyngolaryngeal nystagmus
pharyngolaryngectomy
pharyngomaxillary
    p. fissure
    p. space
pharyngopalatine arch
pharyngopalatinus muscle
pharyngoplasty
pharyngostoma
pharyngotomy
    transhyoid p.

pharyngotonsillitis
pharynx, pl. **pharynges**
phase
    in p.
    opposite p.
    out of p.
    stuttering p.
in phase
phases of stuttering
phenobarbital
    p. with belladonna
phenomenon
    Bell's p.
    Doppler p.
    hesitation p., pl. phenomena
    tip-of-the-tongue p.
    Wever-Bray p.
phenothiazine
phenylbutazone
phenylephrine hydrochloride
phenytoin
pheochromocytoma
pheromone
philtrum, pl. **philtra**
    philtra
phobia
phon
phonasthenia
phonation
    p. break
    hypervalvular p.
    maximum duration of p.
    myoelastic-aerodynamic
      theory of p.
    neurochronaxic theory of p.
    reverse p.
    ventricular p.
    voice disorders of p.
phoneme
    acute p.
    back p.

NOTES

phoneme *(continued)*
- compact p.
- diffuse p.
- front p.
- grave p.
- lax p.
- lenis p.
- segmental p.
- suprasegmental p.
- tense p.

phonemic
- p. analysis
- p. articulation error
- p. regression
- p. synthesis
- p. transcription

phonemics

phonetic
- p. alphabet
- p. analysis
- p. articulation error
- p. context
- p. feature
- p. inventory
- p. placement
- p. power
- p. transcription
- p. variation

phonetically
- p. balanced (PB)
- P. Balanced Kindergarten Word Lists
- p. balanced word (PB word)

phonetician

phonetics
- acoustic p.
- applied p.
- articulatory p.
- auditory p.
- descriptive p.
- evolutionary p.
- experimental p.
- general p.
- historical p.
- impressionistic p.
- p. of juncture
- linguistic p.
- normative p.
- physiologic p.

phoniatrics

phoniatrist

phonics
- vocal p.

phonic spasm

phonogram

phonological
- p. analysis
- p. conditioning
- p. process
- p. process analysis
- p. rule

phonology
- Slosson Articulation Language Test with P. (SALT-P)

phonophobia

phonotactics

phosphatase
- alkaline p.

phosphotungstic acid-hematoxylin (PTAH)

Photo Articulation Test (PAT)

photodynamic therapy (PTD)

photoglottography

photoplethysmographic monitoring

photoradiation therapy

phrase
- carrier p.
- p. structure grammar

phrenic nerve

phycomycosis

phylogenesis

phylogentic change

phylogeny

physiogenic

physiologic
- p. phonetics

physiology

physiotherapy

Piaget's cognitive development stage

PICA
- Porch Index of Communicative Abilities
- posterior inferior cerebellar artery

PICAC
- Porch Index of Communicative Abilities in Children

Picornaviridae

PICSYMS
- picture symbols

pictographs

Pictorial Test of Intelligence

picture
    P. Articulation and
      Language Screening Test
    P. Sound Discrimination
    P. Speech Discrimination
      Test
    p. symbols (PICSYMS)
pidgin
    p. Sign English (PSE)
Pierre Robin syndrome
pigmentosa
    xeroderma p.
pilar cyst
pillar
    tonsillar p.
pi mesons
pink noise
pinna, pl. **pinnae**
    rudimentary p.
piriform, pyriform
    p. aperture
    p. fossa
    p. sinus
pitch
    basal p.
    p. break
    habitual p.
    natural p.
    optimal p.
    p. range
    p. shift
pituitary
    p. gland
    p. tumor
pivot
    p. grammar
    p. word

place
    p. of articulation
    p. theory
placement
    phonetic p.
PLAI
    Preschool Language Assessment
    Instrument
plana
    verruca p.
plane
    cleavage p.
    coronal p.
    fascial p.
    frontal p.
    horizontal p.
    median sagittal p.
    perpendicular p.
    sagittal p.
    transverse p.
planigraphy
planning
    reverse p.
planum
    p. semilunatum
    p. sphenoidale
planus
    lichen p.
plaque
    meningioma en p.
plasma cell
plasmacytoid
plasmacytoma
plasticity
plate
    atresia p.
    bony p.
    bony atretic p.
    cribriform p.
    ethmoidomaxillary p.
    horizontal p.

NOTES

plate *(continued)*
    lateral pterygoid p.
    mandibular p.
    medial pterygoid p.
    metal reconstruction p.
    middle fossa p.
    perpendicular p.
    pterygoid p.
    tegmen p.

plateau
    p. method

plating
    compression p.

platysma
    p. muscle
    p. myocutaneous flap

platysmal

play
    p. audiometry
    p. therapy
    verbal p.
    vocal p.

pledget
    cotton p.

pleomorphic adenoma

pleomorphism
    cellular p.

pleuropneumonia-like organism

plexiform neurofibroma

plexus
    arterial p.
    brachial p.
    cervical p.
    Jacobson's p.
    Kiesselbach's p.
    ranine vein p.
    thyroid p.
    p. thyroideus impar
    tympanic p.

PLGA
    polymorphous low-grade
    adenocarcinoma

plica
    p. semilunaris
    p. stapedis
    p. triangularis

plication
    buccinator p.
    tongue p.

PLOP
    partial laryngopharyngectomy

plosive

plosive-injection method

plucking
    neck p.

plug
    Insta-Putty silicone ear p.
    mucous p.

Plummer bougie

Plummer's disease

Plummer-Vinson syndrome

pluridirectional tomography

plus juncture

PNdB
    perceived noise level

pneumatic
    p. artificial larynx

pneumatized

pneumocephalus

pneumocisternogram

pneumocisternography

pneumococcal infection

pneumoconiosis

Pneumocystis carinii

pneumogram

pneumograph

pneumomediastinum

pneumonia

pneumoniae
    Mycoplasma p.
    Streptococcus p.

pneumonitis

pneumosialosis

pneumosinus dilatans

pneumotachogram

pneumotachograph

pneumothorax

PNS
    peripheral nervous system

pocket
    retraction p.

point
    p. of articulation
    impaction p.
    separation p.

poles

poliomyelitis

poliovirus

Politzer method

pollutant
    air p.

pollution
    noise p.

polyarteritis nodosa

polychondritis
    relapsing p.

polycystic disease
polyfascicular nerve
polyglot
polyglycolic acid suture
polygraph
polymorphemic utterance
polymorphic reticulosis
polymorphous low-grade
  adenocarcinoma (PLGA)
polymyositis
polymyxin B
polyneuritis
    cranial p.
polyneuropathy
polyp
    adenomatous p.
    antrochoanal p.
    nasal p.
    pedicled p.
    pedunculated p.
    vocal p.
polypectomy
    intranasal p.
polypeptide chain
polypoid
    p. degeneration of the true
    fold
    p. hyperplasia
    p. vocal nodule
polyposis
    diffuse vocal p.
    nasal p.
    vocal p.
polypropylene needle
polysyllabic word
polytomography
pons
Pontocaine
pontomedullary junction
Pope wick

Porch
    P. Index of Communicative
    Abilities (PICA)
    P. Index of Communicative
    Abilities in Children
    (PICAC)
port
    nasal p.
    velopharyngeal p.
    p. wine stain
portacaval shunt
portal hypertension
portmanteau word
porus
    p. acusticus
    p. acusticus internus
position
    Boyce p.
    consonant p.
    final consonant p.
    forehead-nose p.
    initial consonant p.
    park-bench p.
    semirecumbent p.
    p. test
    Trendelenburg p.
positional
    p. nystagmus
    p. test
positive
    p. correlation
    p. reinforcer
    p. response
possessive case
possessor-possession
postauricular
    p. area
    p. artery
    p. incision
postcarotid air cell

NOTES

postcentral
    p. gyrus
    p. sulcus
postconcussion syndrome
postconsonantal vowel
postcricoid
    p. carcinoma
    p. squamous cell carcinoma
postdeterminer
posterior
    p. ampullary nerve (PAN)
    p. auricular artery
    p. belly
    p. clinoid process
    p. cricoarytenoid muscle
    p. crus
    p. ethmoid
    p. ethmoidal cell
    p. ethmoidal foramen
    p. ethmoid artery
    p. ethmoid nerve
    p. ethmoid ostium
    p. facial vein
    p. fontanele
    p. fossa
    p. fossa artery aneurysm
    p. incudal ligament
    p. inferior cerebellar artery
      (PICA)
    p. inferior nasal nerve
    p. naris
    p. palatine artery
    p. septal artery
    p. sinus
    sulcus auriculae p.
    p. superior alveolar artery
    p. superior nasal nerve
    p. suspensory ligament
    p. tympanic artery
    p. vertical canal
posterolateral nasal artery
posterosuperior alveolar nerve
postglandular node
postherpetic
    p. neuralgia
    p. otalgia
posticus
    isthmus tympani p.
postlingual
    p. deafness
    p. profound sensorineural
      hearing loss

postnasal
    p. balloon tamponade
    p. drip
postnatal
postpoliomyelitis syndrome
postradiation xerostomia
postresection defect
poststimulus time histogram
posttraumatic amnesia (PTA)
postulates
    conversational p.
postural vertigo
posturography
    dynamic p.
    static p.
postvocalic
    p. obstruent singleton
      omission
potential
    action p.
    auditory-evoked p.'s
    corneoretinal p.
    eighth nerve action p.
      (8AP)
    electrical p.
    p. energy
    nerve action p.
    receptor p.
    vertex p.
potentiometer
    gain p.
    output limiting p.
    threshold kneepoint p.
    variable compression p.
    variable high cut p.
    variable low cut p.
Pott's puffy tumor
Potts-Smith tissue forceps
pouch
    dermal p.
povidone-iodine
power
    p. contralateral routing of
      signals
    p. CROS
    high definition p. (HDP)
    instantaneous p.
    p. peak filter
    phonetic p.
pragmatic
    p. aphasia
    P. Screening Test

p. structure
p. text
pragmatics
preamplifier
pre-article
preauricular
    p. crease
    p. cyst
    p. fistula
precancer
precarotid air cell
precentral
    p. gyrus
    p. sulcus
precession
prechamber
    ethmoid p.
precipitating factor
precision therapy
precochlear cell
preconsonantal vowel
predeterminer
predicate
    p. nominative
    p. objective
    p. truncation
predictive
    P. Screening Test of
    Articulation
    p. validity
predispose
predisposing factor
prednisone
pre-epiglottic space
prefabrication
preference
    consonant-vowel p.
preglandular node
prelacrimal area
prelingual deafness
prelinguistic language

premaxilla
premedication
premolar tooth
prenatal
prenodular swelling
preoperational thought period
prepalate
preparatory set
preparotid fascia
preponderance
    directional p. (DP)
prepsychosis
presbycusis, presbyacusis,
  pl. presbycusi
    stria p.
preschool
    P. Language Assessment
    Instrument (PLAI)
    P. Language Scale
    P. Language Screening Test
    P. Speech and Language
    Screening Test
prescription
prescriptive grammar
presellar
preseptal cellulitis
press
    glossopharyngeal p.
    tongue p.
pressure
    acoustic p.
    continuous positive
    airway p. (CPAP)
    intraneural p.
    intraoral p.
    intrapleural p.
    intrathoracic p.
    minimum audible p. (MAP)
    p. pattern
    pulmonary p.
    p. sore

NOTES

pressure *(continued)*
    subglottic p.
    time p.
presupposition
presyntactic device
pretracheal fascia
prevertebral
    p. fascia
    p. space
    p. space abscess
prevocalic
    p. singleton
    p. voicing of consonant
prevocational deafness
primary
    p. autism
    p. gain
    multiple p.
    occult p.
    p. palate
    p. peak frequency
    p. reinforcement
    p. reinforcer
    second p.
    p. stress
    p. stuttering
principal
    p. clause
    p. vestibular nucleus
principle
    Bernoulli p.
    binary p.
    p. vestibular nucleus
probability curve
probe
    acoustic impedance p.
    blunt lacrimal p.
    hand-held p.
    lacrimal p.
    Reddick/Saye Lav-1
      irrigating and aspirating p.
    p. tube microphone
problem
    gravitational p.
    word-finding p.
procedure
    ablative p.
    Caldwell-Luc p.
    Caldwell-Luc window p.
    canalith repositioning p.
    Cawthorne-Day p.
    commando p.
    Davis-Kitlowski p.

    hypoglossal-facial transfer p.
    inner ear tack p.
    Killian
      frontoethmoidectomy p.
    Language Assessment,
      Remediation, and
      Screening P.
    Lothrop
      frontoethmoidectomy p.
    Lynch p.
    Lynch
      frontoethmoidectomy p.
    modified Weber-
      Fergusson p.
    operant p.
    osteoplastic frontal sinus p.
    Riedel
      frontoethmoidectomy p.
    Shea's p.
    Sistrunk p.
    touch-up p.
    transendoscopic p.
    Weber-Fergusson p.
Procedures for the Phonological
    Analysis of Children's Language
procerus muscle
process
    alveolar p.
    anterior clinoid p.
    ascending p.
    Assessment of
      Phonological P.'s
    auditory p.
    central auditory p.
    Children's Language P.'s
    clinoid p.
    cochleariform p.
    coronoid p.
    developmental
      phonological p.
    feature contrasts p.
    frontal p.
    harmony p.
    lacrimal p.
    lenticular p.
    mastoid p.
    nasal p.
    natural phonological p.
    odontoid p.
    phonological p.
    posterior clinoid p.
    sphenoid p.
    styloid p.

uncinate p.
zygomatic p.
processing
language p.
processor
input signal p. (ISP)
Mini speech p.
output signal p. (OPS)
time domain signal p. (TDSP)
prochlorperazine
production
constricted vocal p.
electrical measurement of speech p.
product moment (r)
Proetz displacement technique
profile
Functional Communication P.
profit
neurotic p.
profound
p. hearing impairment
p. hearing loss
profunda femoris artery
progesterone
prognathic
prognosis
Prognostic Value of Imitative and Auditory Discrimination Test
program
Muma Assessment P. (MAP)
Starkey matrix p.
programmed therapy
programming
articulation p.
progressive
p. assimilation

p. relaxation
p. vowel assimilation
projection
axial p.
coronal p.
coronal oblique p.
frontal p.
horizontal p.
lateral p.
Rungstrom's p.
sagittal p.
Schuller's p.
Stenvers' p.
transorbital p.
projective technique
prolabium
proliferation
clonal p.
lymphoepithelial p.
prolongation
promethazine
prominence
laryngeal p.
promontory
p. stimulation test (PT)
prompt
prompting
pronoun
anaphoric p.
exophoric p.
pronunciation
properant
properdin
prophylactic drug
prophylaxis
proposition
propositional speech
proprioception
proprioceptive
proptosis
propylthiouracil

NOTES

ProSeries laparoscopic laser system
prosodeme
prosody
prostaglandin
prostatic adenocarcinoma
prosthesis, pl. prostheses
    auricular p.
    Blom-Singer tracheoesophageal p.
    Blom-Singer voice p.
    duckbill voice p.
    Panje p.
    partial ossicular p.
    partial ossicular replacement p.
    Singer-Blum p.
    total ossicular p. (TOP)
    total ossicular replacement p.
prosthetic
    p. dentition
prosthodontist
protector
    hearing p.
PROTECT.POINT needle
protein
    iron-binding p.
    perilymph p.
protein-2
    bone morphogenic p. (BMP)
proteinaceous fluid
proteinosis
    lipoid p.
protolanguage
protoword
protracted
protruding ear
protrusion lisp
protuberance
    bony p.
protympanum
provocative food thyroidectomy
proxemics
proxetil
    cefpodoxime p.
proximal
pruritis
Prussak's space
psammoma
PSE
    pidgin Sign English
pseudobinaural hearing aid

pseudobulbar paralysis
pseudocyst
pseudodiverticulosis
pseudoephedrine HCl
pseudoepithelioma
pseudoepitheliomatous hyperplasia
pseudoglottis
pseudohypacusis, pseudohypoacusis
pseudohyperparathyroidism
pseudolaryngeal paralysis
pseudomembranous angina
Pseudomonas
    P. aeruginosa
    P. mallei
pseudomuscular hypertrophy
pseudosarcomatous carcinoma
pseudostratified
pseudostuttering
pseudotumor
    p. cerebri
PSI
    Pediatric Speech Intelligibility Test
psychoacoustics
psychoanalysis
psychodynamic
psychogalvanic
    p. skin resistance
    p. skin response (PGSR)
    p. skin response audiometry (PGSRA)
psychogenic
    p. aphonia
    p. deafness
Psycholinguistic Rating Scale
psycholinguistics
psychometry
psychomotor
    p. seizure
psychoneurological
psychopathology
psychophysics
psychosomatic
psychotherapy
PT
    promontory stimulation test
PTA
    posttraumatic amnesia
    pure-tone average
PTAH
    phosphotungstic acid-hematoxylin

PTD
  photodynamic therapy
pterygoid
  p. muscle
  p. plate
pterygomaxillary fissure
pterygopalatina
  fossa p.
pterygopalatine
  p. fossa
  p. ganglion
ptosis
  brow p.
PTS
  permanent threshold shift
ptyalin
  α-amylase p.
ptyalism
puberphonia
pubic tubercle
pull-through
  p.-t. operation
  p.-t. technique
pulmonale
  cor p.
pulmonary
  p. disease
  p. embolism
  p. function test
  p. insufficiency
  p. pressure
pulsated voice
pulsation
pulse
  alternating p.
  chest p.
  glottal p.
pulsed-current stimulus
pulsed yellow dye laser
pulsion diverticulum

pump
  COMPAT enteral feeding p.
  Gomco p.
  InfuO.R. drug delivery p.
punch
  backward-biting ostrum p.
  side-biting ostrum p.
puncture
  lumbar p.
punishment
pure
  p. agraphia
  p. alexia
  p. aphemia
  p. aphrasia
  p. tone
  p. tone air-conduction
    threshold
  p. tone bone-conduction
    threshold
  p. vowel
  p. wave
  p. word deafness
pure-tone
  p.-t. audiometer
  p.-t. audiometry
  p.-t. average (PTA)
purulent
  p. otitis media
pyoderma
pyogenes
  Streptococcus p.
pyramid
  petrous p.
  truncated tetrahedral p.
pyramidal
  p. eminence
  p. fracture
  p. system
  p. tract
pyriform (*var. of* piriform)

NOTES

Q
 coulomb
quadrangular
 q. cartilage
 q. membrane
quadrant
 anterosuperior q.
quadratus
 q. labii superioris muscle
 q. lumborum muscle
quadrilateral
 vowel q.
quadriplegia
qualifier
quality
 sound q.
quantifier
quantity
 absolute q.

 objective q.
 relative q.
 sound q.
 subjective q.
quartile
Queckenstedt test
question
 tag q.
 yes-no q.
Quickscreen test
Quick Test
quinine
quinsy
quotient
 achievement q. (AQ)
 educational q. (EQ)
 intelligence q. (IQ)
 open q.
 speed q.

R

R
> roentgen

r
> product moment
> roentgen

racemic epinephrine

rad

radial
> r. artery
> r. forearm flap
> r. nerve

radiation
> r. dewlap
> r. therapy

radical
> r. mastoidectomy
> r. neck dissection (RND)
> r. subtotal resection

radicular cyst

radioactive
> r. iodine
> r. iodine uptake test

radiogram

radiograph

radiography

radioimmunoassay

radiolabeled antibody

radiolabeling

radiologic

radiologist

radiology

radionecrosis

radionuclide imaging

radio-opaque dye

radiopaque calculus

radiosensitivity

radiosensitizing drug

radiotherapy

radix nasi

Raeder's syndrome

Rainville technique

Ramsay
> R. Hunt facial paralysis
> R. Hunt syndrome

ramus, pl. rami
> ascending r.

random
> r. flap
> r. movement

r. noise
r. sample

Raney clip

range
> audible r.
> central speech r.
> dynamic r.
> r. of frequencies
> frequency r.
> maximum frequency r.
> most comfortable
> loudness r. (MCLR)
> r. of motion (ROM)
> pitch r.
> sound pressure level r.
> tolerance r.
> vocal r.

ranine
> r. vein
> r. vein plexus

ranitidine HCl

rank
> r. order
> percentile r.

ranula

raphe
> lingual r.
> median longitudinal r.
> palatine r.
> pharyngeal r.

Rapidly Alternating Speech Perception Test (RASP)

rare cleft

rarefaction

RAS
> recurrent aphthous stomatitis

rash
> varicelliform r.

Rasmussen
> fibers of R.

RASP
> Rapidly Alternating Speech Perception Test

rate
> alternate motion r. (AMR)
> r. control
> decay r.
> r. of decay
> r. of maturation
> response r.

ratio
>the oral-nasal acoustic r. (TONAR)
>signal-to-noise r. (S/N)
>s/z r.
>T4/T8 r.

rationalist theory of language
rationalization
raw score
ray
>gamma r.
>roentgen r.

reactance
>inductive r.

reaction
>anticipatory r.
>conversion r.
>dissociative r.
>escape r.
>idiosyncratic r.
>manic r.
>obsessive compulsive r.
>paranoid r.
>r. time

reading
>choral r.
>speech r.

reanimation
>facial r.

reauditorization
rebus
recall
receiver
>air-conduction r.
>bone-conduction r.

reception
>speech r. (SR)

receptive
>r. aphasia
>r. language

Receptive-Expressive
>R.-E. Emergent Language Scale (REEL)
>R.-E. Observation Scale (REO)

Receptive One Word Picture Vocabulary Test (ROWPVT)
receptor
>acetylcholine r.
>antigen r.
>epidermal growth factor r.
>irritative r.

>juxtacapillary r.
>r. potential
>sensory r.
>stretch r.

recess
>elliptical r.
>facial r.
>frontal r.
>pharyngeal r.
>sphenoethmoidal r.
>spherical r.
>tubotympanic r.

reciprocal assimilation
recliner
>Lumex r.

recognition
>oral form r.
>speech r.

reconditioning
reconstruction
>alar r.
>circumferential esophageal r.
>columellar r.
>dermal pouch r.
>epiglottic r.
>hemimandible r.
>mandibular r.
>nasal r.
>neoglottic r.
>orbital rim r.
>ossicular chain r.
>palate r.
>pedicled jejunal r.
>pharyngoesophageal r.
>septal r.
>tracheal r.
>tubular r.

recovery
>spontaneous r.

recruitment
>complete r.
>Metz Test for Loudness R.
>partial r.
>r. test

rectus
>r. abdominis free flap
>r. abdominis muscle
>r. abdominis muscle flap
>r. capitis muscle
>r. medialis muscle
>r. muscle of eyeball
>r. superioris muscle

recurrent
    r. aphthous stomatitis
      (RAS)
    r. bacterial adenoiditis
    r. laryngeal nerve
    r. laryngeal nerve paralysis
    r. respiratory papillomatosis
    r. squamous cell carcinoma
Reddick/Saye Lav-1 irrigating and aspirating probe
reduced screening audiometry
reduction
    alar base r.
    cluster r.
    r. of clusters
    syllable r.
redundancy
reduplicated babbling
reduplication
Reed-Sternberg cell
REEL
    Receptive-Expressive Emergent
    Language Scale
reference
    standard r.
    r. zero level
referent
referential
    r. function
    r. semantics
referred
    r. otalgia
    r. pain
reflected wave
reflex
    acoustic r.
    acoustic contralateral r.
    acoustic ipsilateral r.
    acousticopalpebral r.
    acoustic stapedial r.
    r. arc

    audito-oculogyric r.
    auditory r.
    auropalpebral r. (APR)
    Babinski r.
    cochlear r.
    cochleo-orbicular r.
    cochleopalpebral r. (CPR)
    flexion r.
    gag r.
    gustatory r.
    Hering-Breuer r.
    intra-aural r.
    intra-aural muscle r.
    laryngeal r.
    masticatory r.
    middle ear muscle r.
    Moro's r.
    myotatic r.
    olfactory r.
    orienting r. (OR)
    pharyngeal r.
    round window r.
    sensitivity prediction from
      the acoustic r. (SPAR)
    stapedial r.
    stapedial acoustic r.
    stapedius r.
    startle r.
    stretch r.
    r. time
    trigeminal-facial nerve r.
    vestibular r.
    vestibulo-ocular r. (VOR)
reflux
    gastroesophageal r.
reformulation
refracted wave
refraction
refractory period
regeneration

NOTES

regimen
Furstenberg r.
region
cervicomastoid r.
femoral artery-saphenous
bulb r.
hypervariable r.
parasymphyseal r.
retromolar trigone r.
submental r.
regional
r. anesthesia
r. dialect
r. flap
r. lymph node
r. muscle transfer
register
loft r.
Salivary Gland R.
vocal r.
voice r.
regression
phonemic r.
regressive assimilation
regular determiner
regulator
Ohmeda continuous
vacuum r.
Ohmeda thoracic suction r.
Vacutron suction r.
rehabilitation
aural r.
speech r.
vocal r.
rehabilitative audiology
Reid's base line
reinforcement
differential r.
partial r.
primary r.
r. schedule
reinforcer
conditioned r.
delayed r.
generalized r.
negative r.
positive r.
primary r.
secondary r.
unconditioned r.
Reinke's
R. edema
R. space

reinnervation
Reissner's membrane
relapsing polychondritis
relation
semantic r.
relational word
relations
case r.
relative quantity
relativity
linguistic r.
relaxation
differential r.
progressive r.
r. time
release
Concept CTS Relief Kit for
carpal tunnel r.
laryngeal r.
releasing consonant
reliability
r. coefficient
remission
removal
foreign body r.
hump r.
remover
foreign body r.
remyelination
renal
r. cell carcinoma
r. transplant
Rendu-Osler-Weber disease
REO
Receptive-Expressive
Observation Scale
repair
columellar r.
epineurial r.
repetition
replacement
cervical skin r.
glottal r.
mucosal patch r.
ossicular r.
repositioning
auricular r.
representative sample
repress
repressed need theory
research
comparative r.
resectability

resection
> composite r.
> craniofacial r.
> epidermoid r.
> parotid r.
> radical subtotal r.
> septal r.
> skull base tumor r.
> submucous r.
> transoral r.

reserve
> r. air
> cochlear r.

residual
> r. air
> r. dyskinetic peristalsis
> r. speech
> r. volume (RV)

resistance
> galvanic skin r.
> nasal r.
> psychogalvanic skin r.

resistor

resonance
> r. disorder
> facilitation of r.
> nasal r.
> nuclear magnetic r. (NMR)
> vocal r.
> voice disorders of r.

resonant
> r. frequency
> r. peak control

resonator
> subglottic r.
> supraglottic r.

respiration
> bronchial r.
> cortical r.
> diaphragmatic-abdominal r.
> laryngeal r.

> nasal r.
> opposition r.
> oral r.
> thoracic r.

respiratory
> r. capacity
> r. cilium
> r. disorder
> r. distress
> r. epithelium
> r. frequency
> r. insufficiency
> r. mucosa
> r. syncytial virus
> r. system
> r. tract
> r. tract infection
> r. volume

respirometer
respondent conditioning
responder
> rotation r.
> tilt r.

response
> auditory brainstem r. (ABR)
> auditory-evoked r.
> auditory oculogyric r.
> brainstem auditory-evoked r.
>   (BAER)
> brainstem-evoked auditory r.
>   (BEAR)
> canal resonance r. (CRR)
> catastrophic r.
> conditioned r.
> cortical auditory-evoked r.
>   (CAER)
> covert r.
> delayed r.
> differential r.
> evoked r.
> false-negative r.

NOTES

response *(continued)*
    false-positive r.
    frequency r.
    galvanic skin r. (GSR)
    r. hierarchy
    high frequency r.
    host r.
    immune r.
    late auditory-evoked r.
      (LAER)
    low frequency r.
    r. magnitude
    maladaptive r.
    mean length of r. (MLR)
    middle-latency r. (MLR)
    negative r.
    overt r.
    paradigmatic r.
    positive r.
    psychogalvanic skin r.
      (PGSR)
    r. rate
    slow vertex r.
    somatosensory r.
    r. strength
    syntagmatic r.
    r. system
    target r.
    r. time
    unconditioned r.
    vestibular r.
    vibrotactile r.
restoration
    contour r.
    dental r.
    maxillary r.
restriction
    mandibular r.
restrictive modifier
rest transient
resuscitator
    LIFEMASK infant r.
resynthesis
    binaural r.
retardation
    idiopathic language r.
    mental r.
    perceptual r.
retarded
    mentally r. (MR)
retention
    r. cyst

    linguistic r.
    r. mucocele
reticular lamina
reticulosis
    polymorphic r.
Retin-A
retinal tear
retinitis
retinoic acid
retraction pocket
retractor
    Army-Navy r.
    endaural r.
    Hurd pillar r.
    Jannetta r.
    Johnson cheek r.
    Levy articulating r.
    middle fossa r.
    palate r.
    self-retaining r.
    Senn r.
    Weitlaner r.
retrieval
retroactive amnesia
retroauricular
    r. artery
    r. free flap
    r. vein
retrobulbar neuritis
retrocochlear
retrofacial cell
retroflex
    r. vowel
retrognathic
retrograde
    r. approach
    r. jugular venography
    r. venous drainage
retrolabyrinthine
    r. approach
    r. vestibular neurectomy
      (RVN)
retrolabyrinthine/retrosigmoid
  vestibular neurectomy (RRVN)
retromandibular vein
retromolar
    r. trigone
    r. trigone region
retroparotid lymph node
retropharyngeal
    r. abscess
    r. edema

r. lymph node
r. space
retrosigmoid
r. approach
retrosigmoid/internal auditory canal (RSG/IAC)
retrospective bronchoscopic telescope
retrovirus
reuniens
ductus r.
reverberation
r. room
r. time
reverse
r. phonation
r. planning
r. swallowing
reversibility
Revised Token Test
revision
rhabdomyosarcoma
rheobase
rheumatic
r. disease
r. fever
rheumatoid arthritis
rhinitis
atrophic r.
r. caseosa
r. cholesteatoma
chronic r.
exanthematous r.
hypertrophic r.
r. sicca
r. sicca anterior
vasomotor r.
rhinocerebrophycomycosis
rhinolalia
r. operta
rhinolith

rhinology
rhinophonia
rhinophyma
rhinoplasty
esthetic r.
Rhinorocket dressing
rhinorrhea
caseous purulent r.
cerebrospinal fluid r.
rhinoscleroma
rhinoscleromatis
Klebsiella r.
rhinoscopy
rhinosinusitis
chronic hypertrophic r.
hyperplastic r.
rhinosporidiosis
rhinovirus
Rhizopus arrhizus
rhomboid transposition flap
rhotacism
rhotacized vowel
rhythm
alpha r.
beta r.
delta r.
theta r.
Richard Wolf nasal epistaxis system
ridge
alveolar r.
digastric r.
petrosal r.
petrous r.
superior petrosal r.
supraorbital r.
Riedel frontoethmoidectomy procedure
Riedel's struma
rifampin

NOTES

right
>r. angle bronchoscopic telescope
>r. frontal sinus

right-angle forceps
rigidity
rigid plate fixation
rim
>mandible r.
>r. necrosis

rima glottidis
ring
>Schatzki r.
>targetoid r.
>tympanic r.
>Valtrac anastomosis r.
>Waldeyer's r.

Rinne test
rinse
>oral r.

Risdon incision
risorius muscle
rivinian n.
Rivinus
>R. duct
>notch of R.

Rivinus' notch
RND
>radical neck dissection

Robbins Speech Sound Discrimination and Verbal Imagery Type Test
Rochester method
rodent ulcer
roentgen (R, r)
>r. ray

roentgenogram
roentgenography
Ro intracellular antigen
ROM
>range of motion

Romberg
>R. disease
>R. hemifacial atrophy
>R. sign

rongeur
>Kerrison r.
>Leksell r.

roof
>orbital r.

room
>dead r.

>free field r.
>reverberation r.

root
>r. cyst
>facial nerve r.
>sensory r.
>tongue r.
>r. of the tongue
>r. word

rosacea
Rosenmueller
>fossa of R.
>R. fossa

Rosen needle
rostrum
>sphenoidal r.

rotation
>r. flap
>r. responder
>r. test

rotationally-induced nystagmus
Rotation Test
rote
rotundum
>foramen r.

rough hoarseness
round
>r. forceps
>r. trough
>r. tumor
>r. window
>r. window niche
>r. window reflex

rounded vowel
rounding
>lip r.

Roux-en-Y anastomosis
ROWPVT
>Receptive One Word Picture Vocabulary Test

RRVN
>retrolabyrinthine/retrosigmoid vestibular neurectomy

RSG/IAC
>retrosigmoid/internal auditory canal

rubella
Rubin osteotome
rudimentary
>r. inferior turbinate
>r. pinna

Rudmose audiometer
ruga, pl. **rugae**

rule
    base r.
    morpheme structure r.
    morphographemic r.
    phonological r.
    semantic r.
    sequencing r.
    syntactic r.
Rungstrom's projection
running speech

rupture
rustle
    nasal r.
Rutherford's frequency theory
RV
    residual volume
RVN
    retrolabyrinthine vestibular
    neurectomy

NOTES

sac
> endolymphatic s.
> lacrimal s.

saccade

saccadic velocity test

saccular
> s. collection
> s. cyst
> s. duct
> s. fossa
> s. nerve

saccule
> s. of laryngeal ventricle

sacculus

saddle curve

saddle-nose
> s.-n. defect

sagittal
> s. furrow
> s. incisure
> s. plane
> s. projection
> s. sinus

SAI
> Social Adequacy Index

Saint's triad

SAL
> sensorineural acuity level
> SAL test

salicylate

salience

saline drops

saliva
> submandibular s.

salivarius
> *Streptococcus s.*

salivary
> s. calculus
> s. duct carcinoma (SDC)
> s. duct cyst
> s. fistula
> s. flow test
> s. gland
> s. gland antibody
> s. gland enlargement
> S. Gland Register
> s. leak
> s. lipoma
> s. mucus
> s. peroxidase

> s. pH
> s. test

salivation

salpingitis

salpingopalatine membrane

salpingopharyngeal membrane

salpingopharyngeus muscle

SALT-P
> Slosson Articulation Language
> Test with Phonology

sample
> language s.
> Parsons Language S.
> random s.
> representative s.

Sanders' Venturi injector system

Sandoz nasogastric feeding tube

Santorini
> fissure of S.

saphenous bulb

sarcoidal uveitis

sarcoidosis

sarcoma
> chondrogenic s.
> epithelioid s.
> Kaposi's s.
> mesenchymal s.
> osteogenic s.
> synovial s.

sartoriums muscle

SAT
> speech awareness threshold

satellite nodule

saturation
> s. output
> s. recovery sequence
> s. sound pressure level
> (SSPL)

saucer curve

saucerized

saw-tooth noise

scala, pl. scalae
> s. media
> s. tympani
> s. vestibule

scalded-skin syndrome

scale
> Aphasia Language
> Performance S. (ALPS)

scale *(continued)*
    Arthur Adaptation of the
      Leiter International
      Performance S.
    Cattel S.
    Columbia Mental
      Maturity S.
    developmental s.
    Dos Amigos Verbal
      Language S.
    Hearing Level s.
    Hearing Threshold Level s.
    Minnesota Preschool S.
    Preschool Language S.
    Psycholinguistic Rating S.
    Receptive-Expressive
      Emergent Language S.
      (REEL)
    Receptive-Expressive
      Observation S. (REO)
    sensory s.
    Sklar Aphasia S.
    Smith-Johnson Nonverbal
      Performance S.
    sound pressure level s.
    Stanford-Binet
      Intelligence S.
    Verbal Language
      Development S.
    Vocabulary
      Comprehension S.
    Wechsler Adult
      Intelligence S. (WAIS)
scalenus
    s. anterior muscle
    s. medius muscle
    s. posterior muscle
scalp
    s. flap
    s. muscle
    s. sickle flap
scalpel
    Personna Plus disposable
      Teflon s.
scalping
    s. flap
    s. flap of Converse
SCAN
    Screening Test for Identifying
    Central Auditory Disorder
scan
    CAT s.

scanning
    s. communication board
    scintillation s.
    s. speech
scaphoid fossa
scapular
    s. blade
    s. flap
scar
    hypertrophic s.
    keloid s.
Scarpa's ganglion
SCC
    squamous cell carcinoma
Schatzki ring
schedule
    continuous reinforcement s.
    fixed interval
      reinforcement s.
    fixed ratio reinforcement s.
    intermittent reinforcement s.
    reinforcement s.
    variable interval
      reinforcement s.
    variable ratio
      reinforcement s.
Scheibe malformation
schema, pl. **schemata**
**Schiefelbush-Lindsey Test of
  Sound Discrimination**
Schirmer tear test
schizophrenia
    childhood s.
Schmidt's syndrome
Schneiderian papilloma
Schobinger incision
school language
Schuller's projection
schwa
Schwabach Test
Schwalbe's nucleus
Schwann cell
schwannoma
    acoustic s.
    vestibular s.
Schwartz-Bartter syndrome
Schwartze sign
Sciatic Function Index
science
    communication s.
    hearing s.
    speech s.
    speech and hearing s.

scientific grammar
scintillation scanning
scissors
    Becker s.
    Boettcher tonsil s.
    curved s.
    curved turbinate s.
    curved turbinectomy s.
    Knight nasal s.
    Stevens tenotomy s.
    straight s.
    thin-shaft nasal s.
sclera
    blue s.
scleral shell
scleritis
scleroderma
scleroma
sclerosis
    amyotrophic lateral s. (ALS)
    multiple s.
sclerotic mastoiditis
Scōp
    Transderm S.
scopolamine
score
    Apgar S.
    discrimination s.
    raw s.
    speech discrimination s.
      (SDS)
    standard s.
    word discrimination s.
scoring
    Developmental Sentence S.
      (DSS)
screamer's nodule
screen
    Communication S.
    Communication Abilities
      Diagnostic Test and S.

    Joliet 3-Minute Speech and
      Language S.
screening
    s. audiometry
    S. Deep Test of
      Articulation
    S. Kit of Language
      Development (SKOLD)
    otological s.
    S. Speech Articulation Test
    s. test
    S. Test of Adolescent
      Language
    S. Test for Auditory
      Comprehension of
      Language
    S. Test for Auditory
      Perception
    S. Test for Development
      Apraxia of Speech
    S. Test for Identifying
      Central Auditory Disorder
      (SCAN)
scrofula
scrofulaceum
    Mycobacterium s.
scutum
SCV
    slow-component velocity
SD
    speech discrimination
SDC
    salivary duct carcinoma
SDS
    speech discrimination score
SDT
    speech detectability threshold
    speech detection threshold
sebaceous
    s. adenoma
    s. carcinoma

NOTES

sebaceous *(continued)*
    s. cyst
    s. lymphadenoma
    s. metaplasia
seborrheic
    s. dermatitis
    s. external otitis
    s. keratosis
second
    s. cranial nerve
    cycles per s. (CPS)
secondary
    s. articulation
    s. autism
    s. gain
    s. palate
    s. reinforcer
    s. stress
    s. stuttering
    s. verb
second-look surgery
secretin
secretion
    glairy s.
    viscid s.
    viscous s.
secretomotor fiber
secretory
    s. component
    s. immunoglobulin
section
    frozen s.
sedative
Seddon classification
SEE$_2$
    Signing Exact English
SEE$_1$
    Seeing Essential English
seeding
    iodine-125 s.
    tumor s.
Seeing Essential English (SEE$_1$)
segment
    labyrinthine s.
segmental
    s. analysis
    s. bone defect
    s. mandibulectomy
    s. phoneme
seizure
    jacksonian s.
    psychomotor s.

selective listening
self-concept
self-esteem
self-retaining retractor
self-role concept
self-talk
sellar
sella turcica
semanteme
semantic
    s. aphasia
    s. constraint
    s. feature
    s. implication
    s. relation
    s. rule
    s. theory of stuttering
semantics
    behavioral s.
    extension s.
    general s.
    generative s.
    intention s.
    referential s.
sememics
semiaural hearing protection device
semi-autonomous systems concept
    of brain function
semicircular
    s. canal
    s. duct
semilunar fold
semilunaris
    hiatus s.
    plica s.
semilunatum
    planum s.
semimembranous muscle
semiology
semirecumbent position
semitone
semi-vowel
Semken forceps
semology
Semon-Rosenbach law
Semon's
    S. law
    S. symptom
semustine
senescence
senile
    s. hemangioma
    s. keratosis

senilis
    lentigo s.
senility
Senn retractor
sensation
    s. level (SL)
    s. unit (SU)
sense
sensitivity
    s. prediction from the
      acoustic reflex (SPAR)
sensor
    FLEXISENSOR s.
    s. operation
sensorimotor
    s. act
    s. arc
    s. intelligence period
sensorineural
    s. acuity level (SAL)
    s. acuity level technique
    s. deafness
    s. hearing loss
sensory
    s. acuity level bone
      conduction
    s. aphasia
    s. impairment
    s. nerve
    s. paralysis
    s. receptor
    s. root
    s. scale
sentence
    S. Articulation Test
    s. classification
    complex s.
    compound s.
    compound-complex s.
    constituent s.
    s. constituent

declarative s.
s. derivation
derivation of a s.
derived s.
embedded s.
exclamatory s.
first s.
imperative s.
interrogative s.
kernel s.
matrix s.
nonkernel s.
simple s.
separation
    binaural s.
    s. point
septal
    s. artery
    s. cartilage
    s. perforation
    s. reconstruction
    s. resection
septation
    vertical s.
septi
    depressor s.
septicemia
septoplasty
    frontal sinus s.
septorhinoplasty
    esthetic s.
septum
    bony s.
    deviated s.
    interfrontal s.
    intersinus s.
    intersphenoid s.
    Körner's s.
    mobile s.
    nasal s.
    oblique s.

NOTES

septum *(continued)*
    sphenoidal sinus s.
    tracheoesophageal s.
Sep-T-Vac suction canister
sequence
    inversion recovery pulse s.
    saturation recovery s.
    spin echo pulse s.
    syllable s.
    word s.
Sequenced Inventory of
  Communication Development
sequencing
    auditory s.
    s. rule
sequential memory
sequestrum
    bone s.
serial
    s. content speech
    s. list learning
seriatim speech
seriation
seroma
seromucinous
serosanguineous discharge
serous
    s. cell
    s. fluid
    s. gland
    s. granule
    s. otitis media (SOM)
serratus
    s. anterior muscle
    s. anterior muscle flap
    s. posterior inferior muscle
    s. posterior superior muscle
serum hyperviscosity syndrome
servomechanistic theory
servosystem
Servox
    S. electronic speech aid
    S. Inton speech aid
sessile
    s. lesion
    s. vocal nodule
set
    insufflation test s.
    preparatory s.
    Surgimedics/TMP
      multiperfusion s.
Set-Op myringotomy kit
setscrew

seventh cranial nerve
severe
    s. hearing impairment
    s. hearing loss
sexual characteristics
shadow
    s. curve
    triple line s.
shadowing
    s. method
shape
    syllable s.
shaping
Shapleigh wax curette
Sharplan
    S. laser
    S. Laser 710 Acuspot
SharpLase Nd:YAG laser
sharp loop curette
sharply falling curve
shave excision technique
shears
Shea's procedure
sheath
    carotid s.
    nerve s.
shell
    s. earmold
    scleral s.
shift
    abrupt topic s.
    chemical s.
    Doppler s.
    gradual topic s.
    paradigmatic s.
    permanent threshold s.
      (PTS)
    pitch s.
    temporary threshold s.
      (TTS)
    threshold s.
    topic s.
    voice s.
shimmer
    amplitude s.
shingles
SHM
    simple harmonic motion
shock
    anaphylactic s.
Short
    S. Increment Sensitivity
      Index (SISI)

S. Test for Use with
Cerebral Palsy Children
short-term
S.-t. Auditory Retrieval and
Storage Test (STARS)
s.-t. memory
shower collar
Shrapnell's membrane
shunt
endolymphatic-
subarachnoid s.
Gibson inner ear s.
portacaval s.
tracheoesophageal s.
tracheopharyngeal s.
shunting
electric current s.
Shy-Drager syndrome
sialadenitis
allergic s.
chronic s.
epithelioid-cell s.
granulomatous s.
myoepithelial s.
obstructive s.
suppurative s.
viral s.
sialadenoma papilliferum
sialadenosis
sialagogue
sialangiitis
sialectasis
sialoadenitis
autoimmune s.
bacterial s.
sialocele
sialochemistry
sialogogues
sialography
sialolith
sialolithiasis

sialometaplasia
necrotizing s.
sialopathy
autoimmune s.
sialorrhea
sialosis
sibilant
sicca
s. complex
keratoconjunctivitis s.
laryngitis s.
rhinitis s.
s. syndrome
sickle
s. blade
s. knife
sickness
motion s.
side-biting
s.-b. ostrum punch
s.-b. Stammberger punch
forceps
side-lip forceps
sideropenic dysphagia
siderosis
superficial s.
Siegle otoscope
sieving
mandibular s.
siglish
sigmatism
sigmoid
s. sinus
s. sulcus
sign
Brown's s.
Brudzinski's s. *Hitselberger*
fistula s.
Holman-Miller s.
Kernig's s.
s. language

NOTES

sign *(continued)*
    lipstick s.
    s. marker
    Nikolsky's s.
    Romberg s.
    Schwartze s.
    soft neurological s.'s
    Tinel's s.
    s. word
signal
    s. averaging
    bilateral contralateral routing
      of s.'s (BICROS)
    contralateral routing of s.'s
      (CROS)
    front routing of s.'s (FROS)
    high frequency contralateral
      routing of s.'s (HICROS)
    ipsilateral frontal routing
      of s.'s (IFROS)
    ipsilateral routing of s.'s
      (IROS)
    s. to noise ratio (S/N)
    power contralateral routing
      of s.'s
    square-wave s.
    therapeutic error s. (TES)
signed English
significantly subaverage
Signing Exact English (SEE₂)
SIL
    speech interference level
Silastic implant
silicone
    s. adhesive
    s. granuloma
    s. injection
    s. tube
Silvadene cream
silver nitrate
Silverstein tetracaine base powder
  anesthetic
simple
    s. aphasia
    s. harmonic motion (SHM)
    s. sentence
    s. sound source
    s. syllabic
    s. tone
    s. wave
    s. word
simplex
    herpes s.

simplification
simultaneous
    s. auditory feedback
    s. method
sine wave
Singer-Blum prosthesis
singer's
    s. formant
    s. nodes
    s. nodules
single channel cochlear implant
singleton
    prevocalic s.
singulare
    foramen s.
sinistral
sinistrality
sinodural angle
sinus, pl. **sinuses**
    accessory s.
    branchial cleft s.
    cavernous s.
    dura mater venous s.
    ethmoid s.
    frontal s.
    s. group of air cell
    s. irrigation
    lateral s.
    lateral venous s. (LVS)
    s. line
    maxillary s.
    s. of Morgagni
    paranasal s.
    piriform s.
    posterior s.
    right frontal s.
    sagittal s.
    sigmoid s.
    sphenoid s.
    sphenoidal s.
    straight s.
    s. surgery
    s. thrombophlebitis
    s. thrombosis
    s. tonsillaris
    tympanic s.
sinuscopy
    maxillary s.
sinusitis
    acute frontal s.
    acute maxillary s.
    chronic frontal s.
    chronic maxillary s.

ethmoid s.
frontal s.
maxillary s.
osteoblastic s.
sphenoid s.
vacuum s.
sinusoid
sinusoidal
s. tracking test
s. wave
Sipple's syndrome
Siremobil C-arm unit
SISI
Short Increment Sensitivity
Index
High Level SISI
Sister Helen mustard table
sister-hook forceps
Sistrunk procedure
site
immunocompetent s.
pedicled enteric donor s.
visceral donor s.
six
s. Hertz positive spike
s. Hertz positive spike-
waves
sixth cranial nerve
sixty-cycle hum
sizer
voice prosthesis s.
Sjögren's syndrome
skeleton earmold
skeletonizing
skill
auditory s.
basic s.
Differentiation of Auditory
Perception S. (DAPS)
Test of Auditory-
Perceptual S.

skin
s. expansion technique
s. flap
s. graft
s. island
s. paddle
ski slope curve
Sklar Aphasia Scale
SKOLD
Screening Kit of Language
Development
skull
s. base
s. base tumor
s. base tumor resection
Skytron surgical table
SL
sensation level
slag burn
slang
sleep apnea
slide
slight
s. hearing impairment
s. hearing loss
sling
static s.
temporalis s.
Slingerland Screening Tests for
Identifying Children with
Specific Language Disability
slit fricative
SLN
superior laryngeal nerve
Slosson
S. Articulation Language
Test with Phonology
(SALT-P)
S. Intelligence Test for
Children and Adults
slow-component velocity (SCV)

NOTES

slow vertex response
Sluder
    S. guillotine tonsillectomy
    lower half headache of S.
sludge
slurring
small
    s. cell carcinoma
    s. cup biopsy forceps
    s. fenestra stapedotomy
smallpox
    s. vaccination
SMAS
    superficial musculoaponeurotic
    system
smell impairment
smile
    canine s.
    corner-of-the-mouth s.
    full-denture s.
    Mona Lisa s.
Smith-Johnson Nonverbal
  Performance Scale
Smith & Nephew Richards bipolar
  forceps
smokeless tobacco
smooth muscle antibody
smooth-pursuit eye movement
S/N
    signal-to-noise ratio
snare
    dissection s.
    Tydings tonsil s.
sniffing
sniff method
snoring
snort
    nasal s.
snuff
SO_2
    sulfur dioxide
social
    S. Adequacy Index (SAI)
    s. babbling
    s. behavior
    s. gesture speech
    s. interaction
    s. learning theory
sociocusis
sociolect
sociolinguistics
sodium
    ampicillin s.

    cefuroxime s.
    cromolyn s.
    s. diethyldithiocarbamate
    s. fluoride
    sulbactam s.
soft
    s. neurological signs
    s. palate
    s. palate cleft
    s. tissue window
    s. whisper
soleus muscle
solid-rod rigid telescope
solitarius
    nucleus fasciculus s.
solution
    Burow's s.
    surgical marking s.
    thrombin s.
SOM
    serous otitis media
SOMA
    System of Multicultural
    Assessment
somatosensory response
somesthetic
    s. area
    s. dysarthria
somite
    mesodermal s.
SOMPA
    System of Multicultural
    Pluralistic Assessment
sonant
sone
sonogram
sonorant
sonority
sore
    Oriental s.
    pressure s.
sound
    air-blade s.
    s. analysis
    s. blending
    embedded s.
    s. field
    gross s.
    impact s.
    s. intensity
    s. level
    s. level meter
    non-nasal s.

nonspeech s.
nonsyllabic speech s.
Ohio Tests of Articulation
and Perception of S.'s
(OTAPS)
s. power density
s. pressure level (SPL)
s. pressure level range
s. pressure level scale
s. pressure wave
s. quality
s. quantity
s. spectrogram
s. spectrograph
s. spectrum
standard speech s.
syllabic speech s.
s. wave
sound-symbol association
source
halogen light s.
simple sound s.
xenon light s.
South
S. American blastomycosis
S. American trypanosomiasis
space
air s.
arachnoid s.
buccopharyngeal s.
edentulous s.
fascial s.
lateral pharyngeal s.
paraglottic s.
parapharyngeal s.
peripharyngeal s.
pharyngomaxillary s.
pre-epiglottic s.
prevertebral s.
Prussak's s.
Reinke's s.

retropharyngeal s.
sublingual s.
submandibular s.
submaxillary s.
submental s.
suprahyoid s.
triangular s.
visceral s.
span
attention s.
auditory memory s.
comprehension s.
memory s.
visual memory s.
SPAR
sensitivity prediction from the
acoustic reflex
spasm
chin s.
diffuse esophageal s.
esophageal s.
facial s.
glottic s.
hemifacial s.
laryngeal s.
phonic s.
spasmodic
s. croup
s. dysphonia
s. laryngeal cough
spastic
s. dysarthria
s. dysphonia
s. paralysis
spasticity
spatial balance
spatula
speaker's
s. nodes
s. nodules

NOTES

speaking
    choral s.
specific language impairment
speckled leukoplakia
spectra (*pl. of* spectrum)
spectrogram
    sound s.
spectrograph
    sound s.
spectrum, pl. **spectra, spectrums**
    acoustic s.
    band s.
    sound s.
    tonal s.
speculum
    Cottle nasal s.
    Downes nasal s.
    ear s.
    flat-bladed nasal s.
    s. holder
    nasal s.
speech
    accelerated s.
    s. act
    alaryngeal s.
    s. apraxia
    s. aspect
    Assessment of Intelligibility
      of Dysarthric S.
    s. audiometer
    s. audiometry
    automatic s.
    s. awareness
    s. awareness threshold
      (SAT)
    Bell's Visible S.
    buccal s.
    cold-running s.
    s. community
    compressed s.
    connected s.
    s. conservation
    s. correction
    s. correctionist
    cued s.
    dactyl s.
    deaf s.
    s. defect
    delayed s.
    s. detectability threshold
      (SDT)
    s. detection
    s. detection threshold (SDT)

    s. development
    deviant s.
    s. discrimination (SD)
    S. Discrimination in Noise
    s. discrimination score
      (SDS)
    s. disorder
    displaced s.
    s. distortion
    echo s.
    egocentric s.
    esophageal s.
    figure of s.
    filtered s.
    s. frequency
    s. and hearing science
    high-stimulus s.
    hot potato s.
    hyponasal s.
    s. impairment
    impediment of s.
    s. impediment
    s. improvement
    S. Improvement Cards
    infantile s.
    s. innateness theory
    inner s.
    s. interference level (SIL)
    s. and language clinician
    s. and language pathologist
    s. and language pathology
    s. mechanism
    melody of s.
    mimic s.
    narrative s.
    s. noise
    nonpropositional s.
    parts of s.
    s. pathologist
    s. pathology
    s. perception
    phantom s.
    pharyngeal s.
    propositional s.
    s. reading
    s. reading aphasia
    s. reception (SR)
    s. reception threshold (SRT)
    s. recognition
    s. rehabilitation
    residual s.
    running s.
    scanning s.

s. science
Screening Test for
Development Apraxia
of S.
serial content s.
seriatim s.
social gesture s.
s. sound flow
S. Sound Memory Test
spontaneous s.
subvocal s.
s. therapist
tolerance threshold for s.
s. tracking
s. training unit
tremulous s.
unintelligible s.
visible s.
S. with Alternating Masking
Index (SWAMI)
speech-motor function
speed quotient
SPELT-P
Structure Photographic
Expressive Language Test-II
S-phase specific drug
sphenoethmoidal recess
sphenoethmoidectomy
sphenoid
s. bone
greater wing of s.
lateral wall s.
lesser wing of s.
s. process
s. sinus
s. sinusitis
sphenoidal
s. cyst
s. nasal conchae
s. ostium
s. rostrum

s. sinus
s. sinus septum
s. turbinated bones
sphenoidale
planum s.
sphenoidotomy
sphenomandibular ligament
sphenopalatine
s. artery
s. foramen
s. ganglion
s. neuralgia
spherical recess
sphincter
esophageal s.
eyelid s.
oral s.
spider nevus
spike
diphasic s.
fourteen-and-six Hertz
positive s.
negative s.
six Hertz positive s.
spike-waves
negative s.-w.
six Hertz positive s.-w.
spina helicis
spinal
s. accessory chin lymph
node
s. accessory nerve
s. vestibular nucleus
spindle
s. cell
s. cell carcinoma
spine
anterior nasal s.
s. of Henle
nasal s.
suprameatal s.

NOTES

spin echo pulse sequence
spinosum
    foramen s.
spiradenoma
    eccrine s.
spiral
    s. artery
    s. effect
    s. ganglion
    s. lamina
    s. ligament
    s. organ
    s. sulcus
spirant
spirometer
    Spirometrics Micro & s.
    Timeter pocket s.
Spirometrics Micro & spirometer
Spitz nevus
SPL
    sound pressure level
splayed facial nerve
spleen
splenius capitis muscle
splint
    cap s.
    Gunning s.
    Ultraflex ankle dorsiflexion
      dynamic s.
split
    anterior cricoid s.
    s. calvarial graft
    s. skin graft
    s. word
splitter
    beam s.
split-thickness skin graft
spondee
spondylitis
    ankylosing s.
sponge
    bronchoscopic s.
    gelatin s.
spontaneous
    s. emission
    s. imitation
    s. nystagmus
    s. recovery
    s. speech
sporangia
sporotrichosis
spot
    café au lait s.

    De Morgan s.
    liver s.
spur
    nasal s.
squamous
    s. cell carcinoma (SCC)
    s. epithelial ingrowth
    s. epithelium
square bracket
square-wave signal
SR
    speech reception
SRT
    speech reception threshold
SSL
    subtotal supraglottic
      laryngectomy
SSPL
    saturation sound pressure level
SSW
    Staggered Spondaic Word Test
stabilization
staccato burst
stage
    cognitive development s.
    Piaget's cognitive
      development s.
    stuttering s.
    s. whisper
staged tympanoplasty
Staggered Spondaic Word Test
  (SSW)
staging
    s. system
    TNM tumor s.
    tumor s.
stain
    elastic s.
    Gram s.
    immunoperoxidase s.
    port wine s.
    Ziehl-Neelson s.
stallers
Stammberger punch forceps
stammering
stand
    Mayo s.
    Wilson Mayo s.
standard
    s. deviation
    s. earmold
    s. language
    s. reference

s. score
s. speech sound
s. word
standardization
International Organization
for S. (ISO)
standardized test
standing wave
Stanford-Binet Intelligence Scale
stanine
St. Anthony's fire
stapedectomy
stapedial
s. acoustic reflex
s. artery
s. fold
s. reflex
s. reflex test
stapedis
plica s.
stapedius
s. muscle
s. reflex
s. tendon
stapedotomy
small fenestra s.
stapes, pl. stapes
s. mobilization
s. subluxation
s. superstructure
s. tendon contraction
Staphylococcus
S. aureus
S. epidermidis
Starkey
S. matrix program
S. model ST3 powered
stethoscope
STARS
Short-Term Auditory Retrieval
and Storage Test

startle
s. reflex
s. technique
STAT
Suprathreshold Adaptation Test
state
gradient recalled acquisition
in the steady s. (GRASS)
static
s. acoustic impedance
s. posturography
s. sling
statoconium
Stat-Temp II liquid crystal
temperature monitor
status thymicolymphaticus
steep drop curve
stellate
s. abscess
s. ganglion block
Stenger test
stenosis, pl. stenoses
chronic cicatricial
laryngeal s.
glottic s.
hypopharyngeal s.
laryngeal s.
laryngotracheal s.
subglottic s.
supraglottic s.
tracheal s.
Stensen's duct
stent
laryngeal s.
Stenvers' projection
Stephens Oral Language Screening
Test
steps
branching s.

NOTES

stereocilia
    cochlear s.
    vestibular s.
stereognosis
    oral s.
stereotactic radiation therapy
stereotyped stress
sternoclavicularis muscle
sternocleidomastoideus muscle
sternocleidomastoid muscle
sternohyoideus muscle
sternohyoid muscle
sternomastoid muscle
sternothyroid
    s. muscle
    s. muscle flap laryngoplasty
sternothyroideus muscle
steroid
stethoscope
    Starkey model ST3
      powered s.
Stevens-Johnson syndrome
Stevens tenotomy scissors
stiffness
stimulability
stimulated emission
stimulation
    calibrated electrical s.
stimulator
    electric nerve s.
    Hilger facial nerve s.
    long-acting thyroid s.
      (LATS)
stimulus, pl. stimuli
    conditioned s.
    s. generalization
    neutral s.
    nonpulsed-current s.
    novel s.
    noxious s.
    pulsed-current s.
    s. substitution
    unconditioned s.
stirrup
S&T lalonde hook forceps
stoma, pl. stoma, stomata
stomatitis
    contact allergic s.
    nicotinic s.
    recurrent aphthous s. (RAS)
    s. venenata
stone
    intraglandular s.

stop
    glottal s.
    ubiquitous glottal s.
stopping of fricative
storm
    thyroid s.
Story Articulation Test
Storz equipment
straight
    s. ahead bronchoscopic
      telescope
    s. forceps
    s. scissors
    s. sinus
    s. trough
strain
    eye s.
strap muscle
Strauss syndrome
strawberry
    s. hemangioma
    s. tumor
stream
    breath s.
strength
    s. duration curve
    response s.
Streptococcus
    S. pneumoniae
    S. pyogenes
    S. salivarius
    S. viridans
streptococcus
    β-hemolytic s.
streptomycin
stress
    iambic s.
    s. pattern
    primary s.
    secondary s.
    stereotyped s.
    tertiary s.
    trochaic s.
    s. ulcer
    weak s.
stretch
    s. receptor
    s. reflex
stria, pl. striae
    acoustic s.
    s. presbycusis
    s. vascularis

stricture
    esophageal s.
stridency deletion
strident
    s. lisp
stridor
    biphasic s.
stridulus
    laryngismus s.
string
    initial s.
    intermediate s.
    terminal s.
striola
strip
    fascia lata s.
    packing s.
stroboscope
    Kay's rhinolaryngeal s.
stroke
    glottal s.
stroma
    myxochondroid s.
structure
    base s.
    deep s.
    grammatical s.
    intermediate s.
    language s.
    performative pragmatic s.
    S. Photographic Expressive
      Language Test-II
      (SPELT-P)
    pragmatic s.
    surface s.
    syllable s.
    underlying s.
    s. word
struma
    s. lymphomatosa
    Riedel's s.

Studebaker technique
study
    contrast s.
    electrodiagnostic s.
    immunohistochemical s.
    ultrastructural s.
stump
    nerve s.
stuttering
    cybernetic theory of s.
    exteriorized s.
    hysterical s.
    implicit s.
    incipient s.
    interiorized s.
    laryngeal s.
    laterality theory of s.
    neurotic theory of s.
    s. pattern
    s. phase
    phases of s.
    primary s.
    secondary s.
    semantic theory of s.
    s. stage
    transitional s.
    two-factor model of s.
style
    cognitive s.
styloglossus muscle
stylohyoid muscle
styloid
    s. diaphragm
    s. process
stylomandibular
    s. artery
    s. membrane
stylomastoid
    s. artery
    s. foramen
stylopharyngeus muscle

NOTES

SU
   sensation unit
subarachnoid hemorrhage
subarcuate fossa
subaverage
   significantly s.
subclass
subclavius muscle
subcortical motor aphasia
subcostalis muscle
subcultural language
subcutaneous emphysema
subdigastric lymph node
subdural abscess
subglottic
   s. area
   s. hemangioma
   s. pressure
   s. resonator
   s. squamous cell carcinoma
   s. stenosis
subjective
   s. case
   s. quantity
subjunctive mood
sublabial incision
sublingual
   s. gland
   s. space
subluxation
   stapes s.
submandibular
   s. drainage
   s. duct
   s. ganglion
   s. gland
   s. lymph node
   s. node
   s. saliva
   s. space
submandibulectomy
submaxillary
   s. gland
   s. space
submental
   s. lymph node
   s. region
   s. space
   s. triangle
submentocervical view
submucous
   s. fibrosis
   s. resection

submuscular aponeurotic system
subnasale
suboccipital
   s. approach
   s. triangle
subordinate clause
subperiosteal abscess
subscapular
   s. artery
   s. axis
subsonic
substandard language
substantive
   s. universals
substitution
   s. analysis
   stimulus s.
substitutional lisp
subtotal
   s. cleft palate
   s. glossectomy
   s. laryngectomy
   s. supraglottic laryngectomy
   (SSL)
subtubal air cell
subvocal speech
successive approximation
suction
   s. cannula
   s. forceps
   s. tube
suctioning
sudden drop curve
Sugita microsurgical table
sulbactam sodium
sulcus, pl. sulci
   s. anthelicis transversus
   s. auriculae posterior
   central s.
   s. cruris helicis
   frontal s.
   internal spiral s.
   labial-buccal s.
   lateral s.
   median lingual s.
   paralingual s.
   petrosal s.
   postcentral s.
   precentral s.
   sigmoid s.
   spiral s.
   superior petrosal s.
   temporal s.

terminal s.
s. vocalis
sulfacetamide/prednisone
sulfamethoxazole
trimethoprim s.
trimethoprim and s. (TMP-
SMX)
sulfate
androsterone s.
neomycin s.
zinc s.
sulfur
s. dioxide (SO_2)
s. granule
summation
binaural s.
sump
Argyle silicone Salem s.
Sunderland's classification
Supercut diamond bur
superficial
s. musculoaponeurotic
system (SMAS)
s. parotidectomy
s. petrosal artery
s. petrosal nerve
s. siderosis
s. spreading melanoma
s. temporal artery
s. temporal vein
superior
s. alveolar artery
s. cervical ganglion
s. constrictor pharyngeal
muscle
s. incudal fold
s. incudal ligament
s. laryngeal artery
s. laryngeal nerve (SLN)
s. laryngeal vein
s. mallear fold

s. mallear ligament
s. maxillary bone
s. maxillary nerve
s. meatus
s. nasal concha
s. nasal nerve
nucleus salivatorius s.
s. olivary complex
s. ophthalmic vein
s. orbital fissure
s. orbital fissure syndrome
s. petrosal ridge
s. petrosal sulcus
s. pharyngeal artery
s. pharyngeal constrictor
s. thyroid artery
s. thyroid vein
s. turbinate
s. turbinated bone
s. tympanic artery
s. vena cava syndrome
s. vestibular nucleus
superioris
caput angulare of quadratus
labii s.
levator palpebrae s.
superlative
supermarket vertigo
supernumerary
s. auricle
s. tooth
superstructure
stapes s.
supplemental air
suppletion
support
Dale oxygen cannula s.
Dale ventilator tubing s.
orbital s.
supporting cell of olfactory
epithelium

NOTES

suppression
> failure of fixation s. (FFS)

suppressor-effector T cell
suppressor-inducer T cell
suppressor T cell
suppurative
> s. otitis media
> s. parotitis
> s. sialadenitis

supracarotid air cell
supraclavicular lymph node
supracochlear air cell
supraglottic
> s. resonator
> s. squamous cell carcinoma
> s. stenosis

supraglottitis
supraglottoplasty
suprahyoid
> s. muscle
> s. neck dissection
> s. space

supramarginal
> s. angular gyri
> s. gyrus

suprameatal spine
supramodal perception
supranuclear pathway
supraomohyoid neck dissection
supraorbital
> s. air cell
> s. ethmoid
> s. ridge

suprasegmental
> s. analysis
> s. phoneme

supratentorial approach
Suprathreshold Adaptation Test (STAT)
supratonsillar fossa
supratragal notch
supratrochlear
> s. artery
> s. nerve

supraversion
Suprax
supreme
> s. nasal concha
> s. turbinate
> s. turbinated bone

sural
> s. nerve
> s. nerve graft

surd
surface-coil MRI
surface structure
surgery
> conservation s.
> ear s.
> endoscopic sinus s.
> functional endoscopic sinus s. (FESS)
> laryngeal framework s.
> laser s.
> second-look s.
> sinus s.

surgical marking solution
SURGILASE ECS.01 smoke evacuator
Surgimedics/TMP multiperfusion set
survival
> neuronal s.

susceptibility
suspensory ligament
sustentacular cell
Sutton's disease
suture
> chromic s.
> frontal s.
> mattress s.
> monofilament skin s.
> polyglycolic acid s.
> tympanomastoid s.

SutureStrip Plus wound closure
swallow
> s. method

swallowing
> deviant s.
> infantile s.
> reverse s.
> visceral s.

SWAMI
> Speech with Alternating Masking Index

sweating
> gustatory s.

sweep-check test
swelling
> prenodular s.

swimmer's ear
Swinging Story Test
switch
> compression s.

syllabic
> s. aphonia

complex s.
simple s.
s. speech sound
syllabication
syllabification
syllable
closed s.
s. deletion
deletion of unstressed s.
s. duplication
nonsense s.
open s.
paired s.'s
s. reduction
s. sequence
s. shape
s. structure
sylvian vein
symbiotic
symbol
picture s.
picture s.'s (PICSYMS)
s. set system
Wing's s.
symbolism
symbolization
Visual-Tactile System of Phonetic S.
symmetry
facial s.
sympathectomy
cervical s.
sympathetic vibration
sympatholytic
sympathomimetic
symptom
Semon's s.
vertiginous s.
symptomatic therapy

symptomatology
cerebral palsy s.
synapse, pl. **synapses**
synaptic
syncope
syncretism
syndrome
acquired immunodeficiency s. (AIDS)
Albrecht s.
auriculotemporal s.
Avellis s.
Baillarger's s.
Boerhaave s.
Briquet's s.
Brissaud-Marie s.
callosal disconnection s.
cat cry s.
chromosome 21-trisomy s.
chronic fatigue s.
chronic mononucleosis s.
Collet-Sicard s.
Costen's s.
cri du chat s.
Cushing's s.
Déjérine s.
Down s.
Eagle's s.
Eaton-Lambert s.
Franceschetti's s.
Frey's s.
Gerstmann s.
Gilles de la Tourette s.
Gradenigo's s.
Guillain-Barré s.
Heerfordt's s.
Hunt's s.
hyperkinetic s.
immotile cilia s.
Jackson's s.

NOTES

syndrome *(continued)*
   Kallmann's s.
   Kanner's s.
   Kartagener's s.
   Klinefelter's s.
   Landry-Guillain-Barré s.
   Laurence-Moon-Biedl s.
   Lermoyez' s.
   MacKenzie's s.
   Mallory-Weiss s.
   Melkersson-Rosenthal s.
   Melkersson's s.
   Ménière's s.
   minimal brain
    dysfunction s. (MBD)
   Möbius s.
   mucocutaneous lymph
    node s.
   myofascial pain
    dysfunction s.
   occuloglandular s.
   pain s.
   Parinaud's s.
   Paterson-Kelly s.
   Pierre Robin s.
   Plummer-Vinson s.
   postconcussion s.
   postpoliomyelitis s.
   Raeder's s.
   Ramsay Hunt s.
   scalded-skin s.
   Schmidt's s.
   Schwartz-Bartter s.
   serum hyperviscosity s.
   Shy-Drager s.
   sicca s.
   Sipple's s.
   Sjögren's s.
   Stevens-Johnson s.
   Strauss s.
   superior orbital fissure s.
   superior vena cava s.
   Tapia's s.
   temporomandibular joint s.
   toxic shock s.
   Treacher Collins's s.
   Trotter's s.
   Turner's s.
   Usher's s.
   van der Hoeve's s.
   Vernet's s.
   voice fatigue s.
   Waardenburg s.

synecdoche
synechia
   nasal s.
synechial band
synkinesis
   facial s.
synovial sarcoma
syntactic
   s. aphasia
   s. rule
syntagmatic
   s. response
   s. word
syntax
synthesis, pl. syntheses
   auditory s.
   phonemic s.
synthetic
   s. implant
   s. method
   s. sapphire tip
   S. Sentence Identification
    Test
syphilis
   meningovascular s.
syringe
   Arnold-Bruening s.
   laryngeal s.
   Luer-Lok s.
system
   ABL520 blood gas
    measurement s.
   All Access laser s.
   Allen traction s.
   augmentative
    communication s.
   autonomic nervous s.
   AUTOVAC
    autotransfusion s.
   Barry Five Slate S.
   BiliBlanket phototherapy s.
   Boehringer Autovac
    autotransfusion s.
   central nervous s. (CNS)
   complement s.
   direct motor s.
   dorsalis pedis-FDMA s.
   drainage s.
   Dunlap cold compression
    wrap s.
   endocrine s.
   extrapyramidal s.
   Five Slate S.

Golgi s.
haptic s.
Hopkins rod lens s.
immune s.
indirect motor s.
irrigation s.
Kleen-Needle s.
Mectra
  irrigation/aspiration s.
Modulus CD anesthesia s.
S. of Multicultural
  Assessment (SOMA)
S. of Multicultural
  Pluralistic Assessment
  (SOMPA)
nervous s.
OPMILAS laser s.
Pegasus Airwave pressure
  relief s.
peripheral nervous s. (PNS)
ProSeries laparoscopic
  laser s.

pyramidal s.
respiratory s.
response s.
Richard Wolf nasal
  epistaxis s.
Sanders' Venturi injector s.
staging s.
submuscular aponeurotic s.
superficial
  musculoaponeurotic s.
  (SMAS)
symbol set s.
Universal F breathing s.
Venodyne compression s.
visceral nervous s.
Voice restoration s.
systematic method
systemic lupus erythematosus
s/z ratio

NOTES

NOTES

T
T. cell
T. cell growth factor
T. lymphocyte
T12 nerve division
T4/T8 ratio
T&A
tonsillectomy and
adenoidectomy
tabes dorsalis
table
Andrews spinal surgery t.
Sister Helen mustard t.
Skytron surgical t.
Sugita microsurgical t.
tablet
tabulation
tachylalia
tachyphemia
TACL-R
Tests for Auditory
Comprehension of Language-R
tactile
t. agnosia
t. exteroception
t. feedback
t. kinesthetic perception
t. perception
tact operant
tag question
tail
velar t.
tainting
Takahashi forceps
talk
baby t.
parallel t.
Tall
Lumex Tub Guard T.
tamponade
balloon t.
esophageal balloon t.
nasal t.
postnasal balloon t.
tangible
t. reinforcement of operant
conditioned audiometry
(TROCA)
t. reinforcement of operant
conditioning

TAP-D
Test of Articulation
Performance-Diagnostic
tape
Hy-Tape surgical t.
Tapia's syndrome
TAP-S
Test of Articulation
Performance-Screen
target
t. response
targetoid ring
tarsorrhaphy
task analysis
Tasserit shoulder attachment
taste
t. bud
t. test
tattoo
tautologous
TBG
thyroxine-binding globulin
T-cell count
TD
threshold of discomfort
TDL
temporal difference limen
TDSP
time domain signal processor
teaching
diagnostic t.
tear
retinal t.
t. test
tearing
gustatory t.
tears
artificial t.
crocodile t.
technetium-99m
technique
ascending t.
canal-wall-up t.
communicative t.
cross-facial t.
descending t.
gradient echo t.
head turn t.
high-amplitude sucking t.
(HAS)

technique *(continued)*
    Hood t.
    kinesthetic t.
    lid-loading t.
    masking t.
    Messerklinger t.
    Mohs t.
    Ochterlony gel diffusion t.
    onlay t.
    Orticochea scalping t.
    Proetz displacement t.
    projective t.
    pull-through t.
    Rainville t.
    sensorineural acuity level t.
    shave excision t.
    skin expansion t.
    startle t.
    Studebaker t.
    Terzis t.
    Todd-Evans stepladder
      tracheal dilatation t.
    underlay fascia t.
    Zuker and Manktelow t.
tectorial membrane
teeth (*pl. of* tooth)
    t. malocclusion
    t. malposition
Teflon
    T. injection
    T. mold
tegmen
    t. mastoideum
    t. plate
tegmental encephalocele
telangiectasia
telangiectasis
    hereditary hemorrhagic t.
TELD
    Tests of Early Language
    Development
telegraphic utterance
telephone
    t. booster circuit
    t. ear
    t. theory
telephone-place theory
telescope
    angled t.
    bronchoscopic t.
    0-degree t.
    30-degree t.
    70-degree t.

    foroblique bronchoscopic t.
    retrospective
      bronchoscopic t.
    right angle bronchoscopic t.
    solid-rod rigid t.
    straight ahead
      bronchoscopic t.
telescoped word
Telfa gauze
TEM
    transverse electromagnetic mode
Tempa-DOT single-use clinical
  thermometer
Temple University Short Syntax
  Inventory (TUSSI)
Templin-Darley Tests of
  Articulation
Templin Phoneme Discrimination
  Test
tempo
temporal
    t. arteritis
    t. artery
    t. bone
    t. bone fracture
    t. difference limen (TDL)
    t. fossa
    t. fossa abscess
    t. gyrus
    t. line
    t. lobe
    t. lobe abscess
    t. lobe epilepsy
    t. nerve
    t. sulcus
    t. vein
    t. vessel
temporalis
    t. fascia
    inea t.
    t. muscle
    t. muscle-fascia transfer
    t. muscle flap
    t. muscle transposition
    t. sling
temporary threshold shift (TTS)
temporomandibular
    t. joint (TMJ)
    t. joint syndrome
temporoparietal fascia
tenaculum
    Coakley t.
    White t.

tendency
    bleeding t.
    central t.
tendon
    flexor carpi radialis t.
    flexor carpi ulnaris t.
    stapedius t.
    tensor tympani t.
tense
    t. phoneme
    t. vowel
tension
    t. headache
tensor
    t. fold
    t. tympani
    t. tympani muscle
    t. tympani tendon
    t. veli palatini muscle
tensoris
    incisura t.
tent
    croup t.
tenth cranial nerve
tentorium
TENVAD
    Tests of Nonverbal Auditory
    Discrimination
teratodermoid
teratoid cyst
teratoma
teres
    t. major muscle
    t. minor muscle
terminal
    t. behavior
    clause t.
    t. contour
    t. duct carcinoma
    t. juncture
    t. lag

    t. nerve
    t. string
    t. sulcus
tertiary stress
Terzis technique
TES
    therapeutic error signal
test
    ability t.
    acuity t.
    adaptation t.
    T. of Adolescent Language
    Adolescent Language
    Screening T.
    Allen's t.
    Ammons Full Range Picture
    Vocabulary T.
    aptitude t.
    articulation t.
    T. of Articulation
    Performance-Diagnostic
    (TAP-D)
    T. of Articulation
    Performance-Screen (TAP-
    S)
    audiometric t.
    Auditory Analysis T.
    auditory brainstem
    response t.
    T.'s for Auditory
    Comprehension of
    Language-R (TACL-R)
    Auditory Discrimination T.
    T. of Auditory-Perceptual
    Skill
    Auditory Pointing T.
    Austin Spanish
    Articulation T.
    Bankson Language
    Screening T.
    Barany t.

NOTES

test *(continued)*

Basic Language Concepts T.
t. battery
Bellugi-Klima's Language
Comprehension T.
Berko T.
Bernstein t.
Berry-Talbott Language T.
Bing T.
bithermal-caloric t.
Boston University Speech
Sound Discrimination T.
Brown's t.
California Consonant T.
Caloric T.
Carrell Discrimination T.
Carrow Auditory-Visual
Abilities T.
Cold-Running Speech T.
Competing Sentence T.
Completing Sentence T.
(CST)
Complex Speech Sound
Discrimination T.
could not t. (CNT)
criterion-referenced t.
Culture Fair Intelligence T.
deep articulation t.
Developmental
Articulation T. (DAT)
diagnostic t.
diagnostic articulation t.
Dichotic Consonant-
Vowel T.
Doerfler-Stewart T.
T.'s of Early Language
Development (TELD)
T. for Examining Expressive
Morphology (EEM)
Expressive One-Word
Picture Vocabulary T.
Fein Articulation
Screening T. (FAST)
Flowers Auditory
Screening T. (FAST)
Fluharty Speech and
Language Screening T.
forced duction t.
gaze t.
Glycerol T.
Goodenough draw-a-man t.
Hallpike t.
heterophile antibody t.

Illinois Children's Language
Assessment T.
immittance t.
Iowa Pressure
Articulation T.
James Language
Dominance T.
Kindergarten Auditory
Screening T.
Kindergarten Language
Screening T. (KLST)
lacrimation t.
T. of Language Competence
(TLC)
T. of Language Competence
for Children (TLC-C)
T. of Language
Development-Intermediate
(TOLD-I)
T. of Language
Development-Primary
(TOLD-P)
Language Processing T.
Language Proficiency T.
(LPT)
Lillie-Crow t.
Lindamood Auditory
Conceptualization T.
Lombard T.
maximum stimulation t.
(MST)
Merrill Language
Screening T.
Metz recruitment t.
Miller-Yoder
Comprehension T.
T.'s of Minimal Articulation
Competence
Minimum Auditory
Capabilities T. (MAC)
Monaural Loudness
Balance T. (MLB)
Monothermal Caloric T.
nerve excitability t. (NET)
nonverbal t.
T.'s of Nonverbal Auditory
Discrimination (TENVAD)
T. of Nonverbal Intelligence
(TONI)
norm-referenced t.
Northwestern Syntax
Screening T. (NSST)

Northwestern University Children's Perception of Speech T.
objective t.
ocular dysmetria t.
optokinetic t.
Oral Language Sentence Imitation Screening T. (ORSIST)
Patterned Elicitation Syntax Screening T. (PESST)
Paul-Bunnell t.
Peabody Picture Vocabulary T.
Pediatric Speech Intelligibility T. (PSI)
performance t.
performance-intensity function t.
Photo Articulation T. (PAT)
Picture Articulation and Language Screening T.
Picture Speech Discrimination T.
position t.
positional t.
Pragmatic Screening T.
Preschool Language Screening T.
Preschool Speech and Language Screening T.
Prognostic Value of Imitative and Auditory Discrimination T.
promontory stimulation t. (PT)
pulmonary function t.
Queckenstedt t.
Quick T.
Quickscreen t.
radioactive iodine uptake t.

Rapidly Alternating Speech Perception T. (RASP)
Receptive One Word Picture Vocabulary T. (ROWPVT)
recruitment t.
Revised Token T.
Rinne t.
Robbins Speech Sound Discrimination and Verbal Imagery Type T.
Rotation T.
rotation t.
saccadic velocity t.
SAL t.
salivary t.
salivary flow t.
Schirmer tear t.
Schwabach T.
screening t.
Screening Speech Articulation T.
Sentence Articulation T.
Short-Term Auditory Retrieval and Storage T. (STARS)
sinusoidal tracking t.
Speech Sound Memory T.
Staggered Spondaic Word T. (SSW)
standardized t.
stapedial reflex t.
Stenger t.
Stephens Oral Language Screening T.
Story Articulation T.
Structure Photographic Expressive Language T.-II (SPELT-P)
Suprathreshold Adaptation T. (STAT)

NOTES

test *(continued)*
    sweep-check t.
    Swinging Story T.
    Synthetic Sentence
      Identification T.
    taste t.
    tear t.
    Templin Phoneme
      Discrimination T.
    thyroid suppression t.
    thyrotropin stimulation t.
    Time Compressed
      Speech T.
    Tobey-Ayer t.
    tone decay t.
    topognostic t.
    torsion-chair t.
    Tri-County Contextual
      Articulation T.
    Tuning Fork T.
    Tzanck t.
    University of Pennsylvania
      Smell Identification T.
      (UPSIT)
    vestibular t.
    Visual Aural Digit Span T.
      (VADS)
    Washington Speech Sound
      Discrimination T.
    W-22 Auditory T.
    Weber t.
    Weiss Comprehensive
      Articulation T.
    Weiss Intelligibility T.
    Word T.
    T. of Word Finding (TWF)
    W-1/W-2 Auditory T.
testing
    T.-Teaching Module of
      Auditory Discrimination
      (TTMAD)
testosterone
    t. analog
test-retest reliability coefficient
tetany
    t. neonatorum
tetism
tetracaine
tetracycline
text
    mathetic t.
    nonobtrusive t.

    obtrusive t.
    pragmatic t.
textlinguisitcs
textual operant
thallium imaging
theophylline
theoretical linguistics
theory
    anticipatory and struggle
      behavior t.'s
    approach-avoidance t.
    biolinguistic t.
    breakdown t.
    cerebral dominance and
      handedness t.
    communication failure t.
    conditioned disintegration t.
    diagnosogenic t.
    dysphemia and
      biochemical t.
    empiricist t.
    frequency t.
    frequency-place t.
    Helmholtz' place t.
    innateness t.
    instrumental avoidance
      act t.
    learning t.
    markedness t.
    mixture t.
    nativist t.
    neurochronaxic t.
    operant behavior t.
    perseveration t.
    place t.
    repressed need t.
    Rutherford's frequency t.
    servomechanistic t.
    social learning t.
    speech innateness t.
    telephone t.
    telephone-place t.
    traveling wave t.
    volley t.
therapeutic
    t. error signal (TES)
therapist
    language t.
    speech t.
    voice t.
therapy
    antihormonal t.
    antiretroviral t.

corrective t. (CT)
diagnostic t. (Dx)
interstitial radiation t.
myofunctional t.
neutron t.
neutron beam t.
operant t.
photodynamic t. (PTD)
photoradiation t.
play t.
precision t.
programmed t.
radiation t.
stereotactic radiation t.
symptomatic t.
tongue thrust t.
voice t.
thermal
t. burn
t. noise
thermometer
Tempa-DOT single-use
clinical t.
theta
t. rhythm
t. wave
Thiersch graft
thinking
thin-shaft nasal scissors
thiobarbiturate
thiocyanate ion
6-thioguanine
thiourea
third
t. cranial nerve
t. octave filter
t. projection of Chausse
thoraces (*pl. of* thorax)
thoracic
t. duct

t. nerve
t. respiration
thoracoacromial
t. artery
t. flap
thoracodorsal
t. artery
t. nerve
thorax, pl. **thoraces**
Thorazine
Thornwaldt
T. bursa
T. cyst
T. disease
three-day measles
threshold
absolute t.
acoustic reflex t.
audibility t.
t. audiometry
detectability t.
detection t.
differential t.
discomfort t.
t. of discomfort (TD)
equivalent speech
reception t.
false t.
feeling t.
t. hearing level
intelligibility t.
t. kneepoint potentiometer
noise detection t. (NDT)
pain t.
pure tone air-conduction t.
pure tone bone-
conduction t.
t. shift
t. shift method
speech awareness t. (SAT)
speech detectability t. (SDT)

NOTES

threshold *(continued)*
    speech detection t. (SDT)
    speech reception t. (SRT)
    tickle t.
    vibrotactile t.
throat
    ear, nose and t. (ENT)
    frog in the t.
thrombin solution
thrombophlebitis
    sinus t.
thrombosis
    cavernous sinus t.
    coronary t.
    sinus t.
thrush
thrust
    tongue t.
thumb
    cerebral t.
thymicolymphaticus
    status t.
thymidine
thymoma
thymus
thyration indicator
thyroarytenoid muscle
thyrocervical trunk
thyroepiglottic
    t. ligament
    t. muscle
thyroglobulin
    t. antibody
thyroglossal
    t. cyst
    t. duct
    t. duct cyst
    t. fistula
thyrohyoid
    t. fold
    t. ligament
    t. membrane
    t. muscle
thyroid
    t. adenoma
    t. artery
    t. cartilage
    t. gland
    t. hormone
    t. ima artery
    t. ima vein
    lingual t.
    t. lobectomy

    t. nodule
    t. notch
    t. plexus
    t. storm
    t. suppression test
    t. tissue
    t. vein
thyroidectomy
    completion t.
    provocative food t.
thyroiditis
    de Quervain's
        granulomatous t.
thyroid-stimulating hormone (TSH)
thyroplasty
thyrotomy
thyrotoxicosis
thyrotropin
    t. stimulation test
thyrotropin-releasing hormone (TRH)
thyroxine
thyroxine-binding globulin (TBG)
TIA
    transient ischemic attack
tic
    t. douloureux
ticarcillin
tickle threshold
tidal
    t. air
    t. volume (TV, V_T)
tilt responder
timbre
time
    T. Compressed Speech Test
    t. domain signal processor (TDSP)
    echo t.
    t. pressure
    reaction t.
    reflex t.
    relaxation t.
    response t.
    reverberation t.
    voice onset t. (VOT)
    voice termination t. (VTT)
time-of-flight imaging
time-out
Timeter pocket spirometer
Timoptic ophthalmic drops
TIN
    Tone in Noise

tin ear
Tinel's sign
tinnitus
>t. masker

tip
>CUSA laparoscopic t.
>fiberoptic t.
>nasal t.
>Omni laser t.
>overprojecting nasal t.
>synthetic sapphire t.
>Yankauer tonsil suction t.

tip-of-the-tongue phenomenon
tissue
>abdominal adipose t.
>adipose t.
>angiomatous neoplastic t.
>areolar t.
>cervical soft t.
>collagenous t.
>connective t.
>earlobe adipose t.
>extracapsular t.
>granulation t.
>orbitonasal t.
>peripheral lymphoid t.
>thyroid t.

TLC
>Test of Language Competence
>total lung capacity

TLC-C
>Test of Language Competence
>for Children

TLP
>total laryngopharyngectomy

TMH
>trainable mentally handicapped

TMJ
>temporomandibular joint

TMP-SMX
>trimethoprim and
>sulfamethoxazole

TNM tumor staging
tobacco
>smokeless t.

Tobey-Ayer test
tobramycin
Todd-Evans stepladder tracheal
>**dilatation technique**

Token
>T. Test for Children
>T. Test for Receptive
>Disturbances in Aphasia

TOLD-I
>Test of Language Development-
>Intermediate

TOLD-P
>Test of Language Development-
>Primary

tolerance
>frustration t.
>t. level
>t. range
>t. threshold for speech

toluidine blue
tomography
>computed t. (CT)
>computerized axial t. (CAT)
>dynamic computed t.
>pluridirectional t.

tonal spectrum
TONAR
>the oral-nasal acoustic ratio

tone
>cheek t.
>complex t.
>t. control
>t. deafness
>t. decay
>t. decay test

NOTES

tone *(continued)*
  difference t.
  t. focus
  glottal t.
  modal t.
  T. in Noise (TIN)
  partial t.
  pure t.
  simple t.
  warble t.
tongue
  bifid t.
  black hairy t.
  blade of the t.
  body of the t.
  extrinsic muscles of the t.
  t. flap
  foramen cecum of t.
  forked t.
  t. height
  intrinsic muscles of the t.
  opium smoker's t.
  t. plication
  t. press
  root of the t.
  t. root
  t. thrust
  t. thrust classification
  t. thrust therapy
tongue-jaw-neck dissection
tongue-tie
TONI
  Test of Nonverbal Intelligence
tonic
  t. block
tonofilament
tonometer
tonsil
  t. forceps
  Gerlach's t.
  lingual t.
  Luschka's t.
  palatine t.
  pharyngeal t.
  tubal t.
tonsillar
  t. artery
  t. fossa
  t. pillar
tonsillaris
  sinus t.

tonsillectomy
  t. and adenoidectomy
    (T&A)
  Sluder guillotine t.
tonsillitis
  chronic fibrotic t.
  follicular t.
  hyperplastic t.
  hypertrophic t.
  ulcerative t.
tonsillolith
tooth, pl. **teeth**
  bicuspid t.
  canine t.
  central incisor t.
  cuspid t.
  deciduous t.
  eye t.
  first deciduous molar t.
  first premolar t.
  incisor t.
  lateral incisor t.
  molar t.
  permanent t.
  premolar t.
  supernumerary t.
  wisdom t.
TOP
  total ossicular prosthesis
topical
  t. anesthesia
  t. application
  t. decongestant
topic shift
topognostic test
topography
**Toronto Tests of Receptive
  Vocabulary, English/Spanish**
torque
torsion
  neck t.
torsional wave
torsion-chair test
torsiversion
torticollis
torus tubarius
total
  t. cleft palate
  t. communication
  t. ear obliteration
  t. ethmoidectomy
  t. glossectomy
  t. laryngectomy

Got a Good Word for STEDMAN'S?

Help us keep STEDMAN'S products fresh and up-to-date with new words and new ideas!

Do we need to add or revise any items? Is there a better way to organize the content?

Be specific! How can we make this STEDMAN'S product the best medical word reference possible for you? Fill in the lines below with your thoughts and recommendations. Attach a separate sheet of paper if you need to— *you* are our most important contributor and we want to know what's on *your* mind. Thanks!

(PLEASE TYPE OR PRINT CAREFULLY)

Terms you believe are incorrect:

Appears as: Suggested revision:

_____

_____

_____

New terms you would like us to add:

_____

_____

Other comments:

_____

_____

_____

All done? Great, just mail this card in today. No postage necessary, and thanks again!

Name / Title: _____

Facility / Company: _____

Address: _____

City / State / Zip: _____

Day Telephone No. (   ) _____

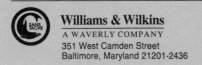

Williams & Wilkins
A WAVERLY COMPANY
351 West Camden Street
Baltimore, Maryland 21201-2436

To order or to receive a catalog call toll free 1-800-527-5597.

#079638-ENT WORDS

t. laryngopharyngectomy (TLP)
t. lung capacity (TLC)
t. ossicular prosthesis (TOP)
t. ossicular replacement prosthesis
touch-up procedure
toxic
t. deafness
t. shock syndrome
toxicity
toxin
botulinum t.
Toxoplasma
T. gondii
toxoplasma lymphadenitis
toxoplasmosis
trachea, pl. **tracheae**
tracheal
t. adenoma
t. agenesis
t. atresia
t. chondroma
t. compression
t. diverticulum
t. fenestration
t. osteochondroma
t. papilloma
t. reconstruction
t. stenosis
t. ulcer
trachealis muscle
tracheitis
tracheobronchial
t. foreign body
t. tree
tracheobronchitis
necrotizing t.
tracheocele
tracheocutaneous fistula

tracheoesophageal
t. cleft
t. fistula
t. puncture dilator
t. septum
t. shunt
tracheomalacia
tracheomegaly
tracheopathia osteoplastica
tracheopharyngeal shunt
tracheoscope
tracheostenosis
tracheostoma valve
tracheostomy
t. tube
tracheotomy
trachomatis
Chlamydia t.
tracing
Bekesy Forward-Reverse T.
I t.
interrupted tracing
interrupted t. (I tracing)
tracking
speech t.
tract
aerodigestive t.
extrapyramidal t.
nasal t.
olfactory t.
pyramidal t.
respiratory t.
upper aerodigestive t.
upper respiratory t.
vocal t.
traction
t. diverticulum
t. headache
traditional
t. analysis
t. grammar

NOTES

tragal
>t. cartilage
>t. notch

tragus, pl. **tragi**

**trainable mentally handicapped
(TMH)**

trainer
>desk-type auditory t.
>frequency modulation
>auditory t.
>hard-wire auditory t.
>Look and Say
>Articulation T.

training
>auditory t.
>discrimination t.
>ear t.
>Language Sampling,
>Analysis, and T.
>visual t.

TRAM flap
>transverse rectus abdominis
>muscle flap

transantral ethmoidectomy

transcanine approach

transcervical approach

transcochlear
>t. approach
>t. cochleovestibular
>neurectomy
>t. vestibular neurectomy

transcortical sensory aphasia

transcription
>broad t.
>close t.
>narrow t.
>phonemic t.
>phonetic t.

Transderm Scōp

transducer

transducing

transduction

transendoscopic procedure

transesophageal varix ligation

transfemoral balloon occlusion

transfer
>dermal fat free tissue t.
>fascia lata t.
>free muscle t.
>hypoglossal-to-facial nerve t.
>intermodal t.
>intersensory t.
>island frontalis muscle t.

linear energy t. (LET)
>masseter muscle t.
>microvascular bone t.
>microvascular free flap t.
>muscle t.
>nerve t.
>pedicled colon t.
>regional muscle t.
>temporalis muscle-fascia t.

transference

transferred meaning

transformation
>malignant t.

transformational
>t. generative grammar
>t. grammar

transformer

**transglottic squamous cell
carcinoma**

transhyoid pharyngotomy

transient
>t. distortion
>t. ischemic attack (TIA)
>rest t.
>t. vibration

transillumination

transistor

transition
>normal t.

transitional
>t. cell carcinoma
>t. papilloma
>t. stuttering

translabyrinthine
>t. approach

transmastoid approach

transmeatal
>t. approach
>t. incision
>t. tympanoplasty incision

transmitter

transmutation

transoral
>t. catheter
>t. resection

transorbital projection

transplant
>alloplastic t.
>renal t.

transplantation

transport
>mucociliary t. (MCT)

transposition
t. flap
muscle t.
parotid duct t.
temporalis muscle t.
Z-plasty t.
transseptal approach
transsexual voice
transtympanic neurectomy
transversalis fascia
transverse
t. arytenoid muscle
t. cervical artery
t. cervical pedicle
t. electromagnetic mode
(TEM)
t. facial artery
t. facial vein
t. plane
t. rectus abdominis muscle
flap (TRAM flap, TRAM
flap)
t. temporal gyri
t. wave
transversion
transversus
t. abdominis muscle
t. linguae muscle
sulcus anthelicis t.
t. thoracis muscle
trap
Lukens t.
trapezius
t. flap
t. muscle
trapezoid body
trauma
dental t.
midface t.
traumagram
facial t.

traumatic
t. granuloma
t. laryngitis
Trautmann's triangle
traveling wave theory
Treacher Collins's syndrome
treatment
ultrasound t.
tree
t. diagram
tracheobronchial t.
Tree/Bee Test of Auditory
Discrimination
tremolo
tremor
essential t.
intentional t.
vocal t.
tremulousness
tremulous speech
trench mouth
Trendelenburg position
trephination
Treponema pallidum
TRH
thyrotropin-releasing hormone
triad
Saint's t.
trial lesson
triamcinolone acetonide
triangle
submental t.
suboccipital t.
Trautmann's t.
triangular
t. eminence
t. fold
t. fossa
t. space
t. vestibular nucleus
t. wave

NOTES

203

triangularis
eminentia t.
fossa t.
plica t.
trichinosis
trichion
Tri-County Contextual Articulation
Test
trigeminal
t. artery
t. nerve
t. nerve artifact
t. neuralgia
trigeminal-facial nerve reflex
trigger zone
trigone
retromolar t.
triiodothyronine
trill
Trilogy I hearing aid
trim
freeze t.
trimalar fracture
trimethoprim
t. and sulfamethoxazole
(TMP-SMX)
t. sulfamethoxazole
trimetrexate
triphosphate
adenosine t. (ATP)
triphthong
triplegia
triple line shadow
tripod fracture
trismus
trite
triticea
cartilago t.
TROCA
tangible reinforcement of
operant conditioned
audiometry
trocar
Hasson laparoscopic t.
trochaic stress
trochlear nerve
Trolard
vein of T.
Trotter's syndrome
trough
t. curve
round t.
straight t.

true
t. language
t. vocal fold
truncated tetrahedral pyramid
truncation
predicate t.
trunk
cervicofacial t.
nerve t.
thyrocervical t.
trypanosomiasis
South American t.
TSH
thyroid-stimulating hormone
TSTI
tumor-specific transplantation
immunity
TTMAD
Testing-Teaching Module of
Auditory Discrimination
TTS
temporary threshold shift
tubal
t. catarrh
t. tonsil
tubarius
torus t.
tube
aspiration t.
auditory t.
Baker self-sumping t.
Donaldson t.
double-cannula
tracheostomy t.
double-lumen suction
irrigation t.
endoneurial t.
endotracheal t.
eustachian t.
t. extrusion
feeding t.
gastrostomy feeding t.
Heimlich t.
Kangaroo gastrostomy
feeding t.
Lukens collecting t.
Moss balloon triple-lumen
gastrostomy t.
nasogastric t.
Sandoz nasogastric
feeding t.
silicone t.
suction t.

tracheostomy t.
tympanotomy t.
ventilation t.
Wolf suction t.
tubercle
Darwin's t.
epiglottic t.
pubic t.
Whitnall's t.
tuberculoma
tuberculosis
Mycobacterium t.
tuberculous
t. adenitis
t. otitis media
tuberculum
tubotympanic recess
tubular reconstruction
Tucker
T. bougie
T. mediastinoscope
T. staple forceps
T. tack and pin forceps
tularemia
tularensis
Francisella t.
tumor
acinic cell t.
adenoid cystic t.
aerodigestive t.
basaloid t.
benign mixed t.
brain t.
Brooke's t.
t. burden
t. capsule
cerebellopontine angle t.
deep-lobe t.
dermal analogue t.
eighth nerve t.
epidermoid t.

giant cell t.
glomus t.
glomus jugulare t.
glomus tympanicum t.
glomus vagale t.
t. imaging
intracranial t.
keloid t.
lymphoreticular t.
t. marker
mesenchymal t.
metachronous t.
mucoepidermoid t.
nerve sheath t.
neurogenic t.
petrous apex t.
pituitary t.
Pott's puffy t.
round t.
t. seeding
skull base t.
t. stage grouping
t. staging
strawberry t.
turban t.
vascular t.
vasoformative t.
Warthin's t.
tumor-specific
t.-s. antigen
t.-s. transplantation
immunity (TSTI)
tunable
t. notch filter
t. tinnitus masker
tuneable dye laser
tuning
cochlear t.
t. curve
T. Fork Test
tunnel of Corti

NOTES

turban tumor
turbinate
    inferior t.
    middle t.
    neck of middle t.
    paradoxic t.
    rudimentary inferior t.
    superior t.
    supreme t.
turbinated bones
turbinectomy
turbinoplasty
turbulence
    nasal t.
turcica
    sella t.
Turner's syndrome
TUSSI
    Temple University Short Syntax
    Inventory
TV
    tidal volume
twang
    nasal t.
twelfth cranial nerve
TWF
    Test of Word Finding
twin language
twist
    t. drill
    octave t.
two-factor model of stuttering
two-team dissection
two-toned voice
Tycos pressure infusion line
Tydings tonsil snare
tympani
    canaliculus of chorda t.
    chorda t.
    scala t.
    tensor t.
tympanic
    t. annulus

    t. artery
    t. cavity
    t. cell
    t. fold
    t. homograft
    t. membrane
    t. muscle
    t. nerve
    t. neurectomy
    t. plexus
    t. ring
    t. sinus
tympanica
    incisura t.
tympanicus
    annulus t.
tympanitis
tympanogram
    t. classification (Feldman
    model)
    t. classification (Jerger
    model)
tympanomastoid
    t. fissure
    t. suture
tympanomastoidectomy
tympanomeatal flap
tympanometry
tympanoplasty
    t. mastoidectomy
    t. ossiculoplasty
    staged t.
tympanosclerosis
tympanosclerotic
tympanotomy
    t. tube
types
    Bekesy tracing t.
tyrosine crystal
tyrothricin
Tzanck test

ubiquitous glottal stop
UCL
    uncomfortable level
    uncomfortable loudness level
UICC
    Union Internationale Contre
    Cancrum
ulcer
        Barrett's u.
        contact u.
        Cushing u.
        duodenal u.
        oropharyngeal u.
        peptic u.
        rodent u.
        stress u.
        tracheal u.
ulceration
        corneal u.
ulcerative
        u. gingivitis
        u. tonsillitis
Ultraflex ankle dorsiflexion
    dynamic splint
UltraLine Nd:YAG laser fiber
UltraPulse surgical laser
ultrasonic
        u. frequency
ultrasonography
ultrasound-guided biopsy
ultrasound treatment
ultrastructural study
ULTRA ultrasonic aspirator
umbo
unaided augmentative
    communication
Unasyn
uncinate process
uncinectomy
uncomfortable
        u. level (UCL)
        u. loudness level (UCL)
unconditioned
        u. reinforcer
        u. response
        u. stimulus
uncoupling
        nasal u.
underbite
underextension

underlay fascia technique
underlying structure
undermasking
undifferentiated carcinoma
undulant fever
unilateral
        u. abductor paralysis
        u. adductor paralysis
        u. cleft lip
        u. cleft palate
        u. hearing loss
        u. paralysis
        u. weakness
unilocular
unimodal
unintelligible speech
Union Internationale Contre
    Cancrum (UICC)
unipedicled flap
unisensory
unit
        auditory training u.'s
        Hounsfield u.
        loudness u.
        Ohmeda intermittent
          suction u.
        osteomeatal u.
        ostiomeatal u. (OMU)
        sensation u. (SU)
        Siremobil C-arm u.
        speech training u.
United States of America
    Standards Institute (USASI)
Universal
        U. F breathing system
universal grammar
universality
universals
        formal u.
        linguistic u.
        substantive u.
University of Pennsylvania Smell
    Identification Test (UPSIT)
unmitigated echolalia
unresectable squamous cell
    carcinoma
unrounded vowel
unstressed
        u. syllable deletion
        u. vowel

upbiting forceps
upper
    u. aerodigestive tract
    u. airway
    u. airway obstruction
    u. bound
    u. cervical nerve
    u. lateral cartilage
    u. lateral nasal cartilage
    u. partial
    u. respiratory infection
     (URI)
    u. respiratory tract
    u. respiratory tract infection
    u. trapezius flap
UPSIT
    University of Pennsylvania
    Smell Identification Test
upturned forceps
upward
    u. bent forceps
    u. masking
uranoplasty
uranoschisis
Urecholine
uremia
URI
    upper respiratory infection
usage doctrine

USASI
    United States of America
    Standards Institute
U-shaped
    U.-s. curve
    U.-s. incision
Usher's syndrome
Utah Test of Language
    Development
utricle
utricular duct
utriculoendolymphatic valve
utriculosaccular duct
utriculus
utterance
    holophrastic u.
    mean length of u. (MLU)
    mean relational u. (MRU)
    polymorphemic u.
    telegraphic u.
uveitis
    sarcoidal u.
uveoparotid fever
uvula
uvular
    u. muscle
uvulopalatopharyngoplasty
uvulopharyngeal

V_T
 tidal volume
vaccination
 smallpox v.
 variola v.
vaccine
Vaccinia
Vacu-Irrigator
 Lap V.-I.
vacuolation
Vacutron suction regulator
vacuum sinusitis
VADS
 Visual Aural Digit Span Test
vaginal process of the sphenoid
 bone
vagotomy
vagus nerve
validity
 concurrent v.
 construct v.
 content v.
 criterion related v.
 face v.
 predictive v.
Valium
vallate papilla
vallecula, pl. valleculae
Valsalva maneuver
Valtrac anastomosis ring
valve
 anterior nasal v.
 Argyle anti-reflux v.
 nasal v.
 tracheostoma v.
 utriculoendolymphatic v.
 velopharyngeal v.
valves of Kerckring
van der Hoeve's syndrome
Vantin
vaporization
variable
 v. compression
  potentiometer
 v. high cut potentiometer
 v. interval reinforcement
  schedule
 v. low cut potentiometer

v. ratio reinforcement
 schedule
v. release compression
variation
 free v.
 linguistic v.
 phonetic v.
varicella
varicella-zoster encephalitis
varicelliform rash
varices (*pl. of* varix)
variegated pattern
variola
 v. vaccination
varix, pl. varices
 esophageal v.
vascular
 v. endothelium
 v. headache
 v. malformation
 v. pedicle
 v. tumor
vascularis
 stria v.
vasoconstriction
vasoconstrictive agent
vasoconstrictor
vasodilator
vasoformative tumor
vasomotor rhinitis
vasonervorum
vasospasm
Vater
 papilla of V.
VC
 vital capacity
V-C
 vowel-consonant
vegetans
 pemphigus v.
vein
 angular v.
 angular facial v.
 anterior facial v.
 auditory v.
 axillary v.
 cerebellar v.
 cochlear v.
 common facial v.
 condylar emissary v.

vein *(continued)*
    cortical v.
    emissary v.
    external jugular v.
    facial v.
    inferior thyroid v.
    internal auditory v.
    internal jugular v.
    jugular v.
    v. of Labbé
    laryngeal v.
    mastoid emissary v.
    maxillary v.
    middle thyroid v.
    pharyngeal v.
    posterior facial v.
    ranine v.
    retroauricular v.
    retromandibular v.
    superficial temporal v.
    superior laryngeal v.
    superior ophthalmic v.
    superior thyroid v.
    sylvian v.
    temporal v.
    thyroid v.
    thyroid ima v.
    transverse facial v.
    v. of Trolard
vela *(pl. of* velum)
velar
    v. area
    v. assimilation
    backing to v.
    v. insufficiency
    v. tail
velarized consonant
velocity
    particle v.
    slow-component v. (SCV)
velopharyngeal
    v. closure
    v. competence
    v. incompetence
    v. insufficiency
    v. port
    v. valve
velum, pl. vela
    v. palati
venae comitantes
venenata
    dermatitis v.
    stomatitis v.

Venodyne compression system
venography
    jugular v.
    retrograde jugular v.
vent
vented earmold
ventilation
    cuirass v.
    v. tube
    v. tube inserter
ventral
ventricle
    appendix of laryngeal v.
    laryngeal v.
    v. of Morgagni
    saccule of laryngeal v.
ventricular
    v. dysphonia
    v. fold
    v. phonation
ventriculocordectomy
ventriculus laryngis
ventroposteriorinferior nucleus
verb
    auxiliary v.
    helping v.
    linking v.
    secondary v.
verbal
    v. aphasia
    v. apraxia
    v. fluency
    V. Language Development
      Scale
    v. mediation
    v. operant
    v. paraphrasia
    v. play
verbigeration
verbotonal method
vermilion
    v. border
vernacular
Vernet's syndrome
Verocay body
verruca
    v. plana
    v. vulgaris
verrucous carcinoma
vertebral artery
vertebral-basilar artery disease
vertex potential

vertical
    v. crest
    v. lip biopsy
    v. septation
verticalis linguae muscle
vertiginous symptom
vertigo
    benign paroxysmal
      positional v. (BPPV)
    benign positional v. (BPV)
    cervical v.
    laryngeal v.
    paroxysmal positional v.
    postural v.
    supermarket v.
vesicle
    olfactory v.
    otic v.
vessel
    blood v.
    circumflex scapular v.
    friable v.
    intercostal v.
    mucosal blood v.
    temporal v.
vestibula (*pl. of* vestibulum)
vestibular
    v. apparatus
    v. aqueduct
    v. canal
    v. cecum
    v. fold
    v. fossa
    v. ganglion
    v. hydrops
    v. labyrinth
    v. ligament
    v. membrane
    v. nerve
    v. neurectomy (VN)

    v. neuritis
    v. neuronitis
    v. nucleus
    v. nystagmus
    v. pathway
    v. reflex
    v. response
    v. schwannoma
    v. stereocilia
    v. test
    v. window
vestibule
    laryngeal v.
    nasal v.
vestibuli (*gen. of* vestibulum)
vestibulitis
    nasal v.
vestibulocerebellar connection
vestibulocerebellum
vestibulocochlear
    v. artery
    v. nerve
vestibulofibrosis
vestibulo-infraglottic duct
vestibulometry
vestibulo-ocular reflex (VOR)
vestibulum, gen. **vestibuli**,
   pl. **vestibula**
    scala vestibuli
vibrant consonant
vibration
    forced v.
    free v.
    glottal v.
    v. meter
    sympathetic v.
    transient v.
vibrato
vibrator
    bone-conduction v.

NOTES

vibratory cycle
vibrissa, pl. **vibrissae**
    nasal v.
vibrometer
vibrotactile
    v. hearing aid
    v. response
    v. threshold
Vicous
Video-fluoroscopic imaging chair
video monitoring
videostrobe
videostroboscopy
vidian
    v. artery
    v. canal
    v. nerve
view
    Caldwell v.
    chin-nose v.
    jug-handle v.
    laryngoscopic v.
    Mayer's v.
    occipitomeatal v.
    Owen's v.
    submentocervical v.
    Waters v.
vinblastine
Vincent's angina
vincristine
violet
    Gentian v.
viral
    v. infection
    v. labyrinthitis
    v. sialadenitis
virgules
viridans
    Streptococcus v.
virilization
virus
    ECHO v.
    enterocytopathogenic human
      orphan v.
    Epstein-Barr v. (EBV)
    herpes v.
    human immunodeficiency v.
      (HIV)
    human T cell
      lymphotrophic v. (HTLV)
    influenza A v.
    lymphadenopathy-
      associated v. (LAV)

    lymphocyte-associated v.
      (LAV)
    parainfluenza v.
    respiratory syncytial v.
VISA multi-patient monitor
viscera (*pl. of* viscus)
visceral
    v. donor site
    v. fascia
    v. nervous system
    v. space
    v. swallowing
viscid secretion
viscosity
viscous secretion
viscus, pl. **viscera**
visible speech
Visi-pitch
visor
    v. angle
    v. flap
visual
    v. acuity
    v. agnosia
    v. alexia
    v. area
    V. Aural Digit Span Test
      (VADS)
    v. closure
    v. cue
    v. discrimination
    v. figure-ground
    v. figure-ground
      discrimination
    v. memory
    v. memory span
    v. method
    v. perception
    V. Reinforcement
      Audiometry
    v. training
visual-motor
    v.-m. coordination
    v.-m. function
Visual-Tactile System of Phonetic
  Symbolization
visual-verbal agnosia
vital capacity (VC)
vitamin
    v. A deficiency
    v. B deficiency
    v. deficiency
vitreous cavity

**V-Lok disposable blood
 pressure cuff**
VN
 vestibular neurectomy
vocabulary
 V. Comprehension Scale
 core v.
vocal
 v. abuse
 v. attack
 v. band
 v. capability battery
 v. constriction
 v. cord
 v. cord bowing
 v. cord injection
 v. cord nodule
 v. cord paralysis
 v. efficiency
 v. effort
 v. fatigue
 v. focus
 v. fold
 v. fold approximation
 v. fold paralysis
 v. fry
 v. ligament
 v. misuse
 v. mode
 v. muscle
 v. nodule
 v. organ
 v. phonics
 v. play
 v. polyp
 v. polyposis
 v. range
 v. register
 v. rehabilitation
 v. resonance

 v. tract
 v. tremor
vocalic
 v. glide
vocalis
 v. muscle
 sulcus v.
vocalization
voice
 active v.
 adolescent v.
 v. building
 chest v.
 v. clinician
 v. disorder
 v. disorders of phonation
 v. disorders of resonance
 esophageal v.
 eunuchoid v.
 falsetto v.
 v. fatigue
 v. fatigue syndrome
 gravel v.
 guttural v.
 inspiratory v.
 light v.
 muffled v.
 mutation v.
 v. onset time (VOT)
 passive v.
 v. pathologist
 v. prosthesis sizer
 pulsated v.
 v. register
 V. restoration system
 v. shift
 v. termination time (VTT)
 v. therapist
 v. therapy
 v. tone focus

NOTES

voice *(continued)*
    transsexual v.
    two-toned v.
voiced
    v. consonant
voiceless
    v. consonant
voicing
    consonant v.
volition
    v. oral movement
volley theory
volt
volume
    v. control
    expiratory reserve v. (ERV)
    forced expiratory v. (FEV)
    inspiratory reserve v. (IRV)
    lung v.
    residual v. (RV)
    respiratory v.
    tidal v. (TV, V_T)
    v. unit meter (VU meter)
voluntary mutism
vomer
vomeronasal
    v. cartilage
    v. organ
von
    v. Ebner's gland
    v. Frisch bacillus
    v. Recklinghausen's disease
VOR
    vestibulo-ocular reflex
VOT
    voice onset time
vowel
    back v.
    cardinal v.

central v.
close v.
front v.
high v.
indefinite v.
interconsonantal v.
lax v.
light v.
low v.
mid v.
narrow v.
nasalization of v.
neutral v.
v. neutralization
obscure v.
open v.
postconsonantal v.
preconsonantal v.
pure v.
v. quadrilateral
retroflex v.
rhotacized v.
rounded v.
tense v.
unrounded v.
unstressed v.
vowel-consonant (V-C)
vowelization
VP16-213
VTT
    voice termination time
vu
    déjà v.
vulgaris
    lupus v.
    pemphigus v.
    verruca v.
VU meter

W-1/W-2 Auditory Test
W-22 Auditory Test
Waardenburg syndrome
WAB
  Western Aphasia Battery
Wadenstrom's macroglobulinemia
WAIS
  Wechsler Adult Intelligence
  Scale
Waldeyer's ring
wall
  infratemporal w.
  perpendicular anterior w.
Wallerian degeneration
warble tone
warm-wire anemometer
wart
Warthin's
  W. area
  W. tumor
Warthin-Starry staining method
Washington Speech Sound
  Discrimination Test
wastage
  air w.
waterfall curve
Waters view
watertight closure
Watson duckbill forceps
watt
wave
  alpha w.
  aperiodic w.
  beta w.
  complex w.
  cosine w.
  damped w.
  delta w.
  diffracted w.
  electromagnetic w.
  w. filter
  incident w.
  longitudinal w.
  nonperiodic w.
  notched w.
  periodic w.
  pure w.
  reflected w.
  refracted w.

simple w.
sine w.
sinusoidal w.
sound w.
sound pressure w.
standing w.
theta w.
torsional w.
transverse w.
triangular w.
waveform
  w. distortion
wavelength
waveshape
wax
  bone w.
  w. curette
weak
  w. stress
  w. syllable deletion
weakness
  unilateral w.
web
  esophageal w.
  laryngeal w.
webbing
Weber-Fergusson procedure
Weber test
Webster needle holder
Wechsler
  W. Adult Intelligence Scale
  (WAIS)
  W. Intelligence Scale for
  Children-Revised (WISC-R)
  W. Preschool and Primary
  Scale of Intelligence
  (WPPSI)
Weerda distending operating
  laryngoscope
Wegener's granulomatosis
weight loss
Weimert epistaxis packing
Weiss
  W. Comprehensive
  Articulation Test
  W. Intelligibility Test
Weitlaner retractor
wens

Wernicke's
  W. aphasia
  W. area
Western Aphasia Battery (WAB)
wet hoarseness
Wever-Bray
  W.-B. effect
  W.-B. phenomenon
Wharton's duct
whirlybird
whisper
  buccal w.
  soft w.
  stage w.
whispering
  involuntary w.
white
  w. dural fold
  w. noise
  w. sponge lesion of Cannon
White tenaculum
Whitnall's tubercle
Whorf's hypothesis
wick
  Pope w.
wide-band noise
wide-field total laryngectomy
wide range audiometer
Wilde ethmoid forceps
Willis
  circle of W.
willisiana
  paracusia w.
Willis' paracusis
Wilson Mayo stand
window
  cochlear w.
  lung w.
  nasoantral w.
  oval w.
  round w.
  soft tissue w.
  vestibular w.
windpipe
Wing's symbol
Winkler's disease
WIPI
  Word Intelligibility by Picture
  Identification
wire
  interosseous w.

WISC-R
  Wechsler Intelligence Scale for
  Children-Revised
wisdom tooth
Wolf
  W. equipment
  W. suction tube
**Woodcock Language Proficiency
Battery, English Form**
word
  ambiguous w.
  w. approximation
  w. association
  base w.
  w. blindness
  w. calling
  class w.
  w. class
  clipped w.
  complex w.
  compound w.
  w. configuration
  content w.
  contentive w.
  w. count
  w. deafness
  w. discrimination score
  feared w.
  first w.
  form w.
  function w.
  heterogeneous w.
  homogenous w.
  W. Intelligibility by Picture
  Identification (WIPI)
  interstitial w.
  Jonah w.
  lexical w.
  monosyllabic w.
  nonsense w.
  open w.
  paradigmatic w.
  PB w.
    phonetically balanced word
  phonetically balanced w.
  (PB word)
  pivot w.
  polysyllabic w.
  portmanteau w.
  relational w.
  root w.
  w. sequence
  sign w.

simple w.
split w.
standard w.
structure w.
syntagmatic w.
telescoped w.
W. Test
word-finding problem
worker's compensation
wound
   w. care

gunshot w. (GSW)
   w. infection
   w. necrosis
WPPSI
   Wechsler Preschool and Primary
   Scale of Intelligence
Wrisberg
   cuneiform cartilage of W.
Wrisberg's cartilage
written language

NOTES

X

xenon light source
xeroderma pigmentosa
xerography
xeroradiogram

xerostomia
    postradiation x.
x-ray
Xylocaine

X

Yankauer tonsil suction tip
yawn-sigh approach
Y-cord hearing aid

yes-no question
Y incision
Y-port connector

Y

Zeiss
> Z. microscope
> Z. operating microscope

Zelco Flexlite
zellballen
Zenker's diverticulum
zero
> z. amplitude
> audiometric z.
> z. cerebral
> z. hearing level
> z. morpheme

Ziehl-Neelson stain
Zimmer clip
Zinacef
zinc sulfate
zone
> trigger z.

zoster
> herpes z.

Zovirax
Z-plasty
> Z.-p. transposition

Zuker and Manktelow technique
zygoma
zygomal cell
zygomatic
> z. arch
> z. bone
> z. branch
> z. fracture
> z. frontal nerve
> z. osteomyelitis
> z. process
> z. temporal nerve

zygomaticus
> z. major muscle
> z. muscle

Zymogen granule

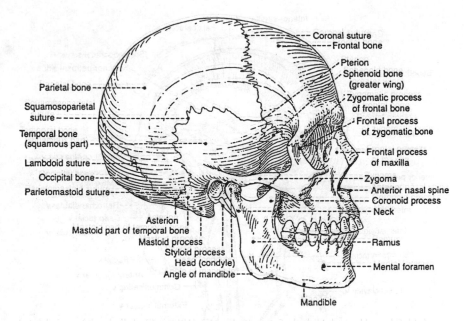

Lateral view of the skull. In Chung KW. Gross Anatomy, 2nd ed. Malvern, Harwal Publishing, 1991.

Appendices

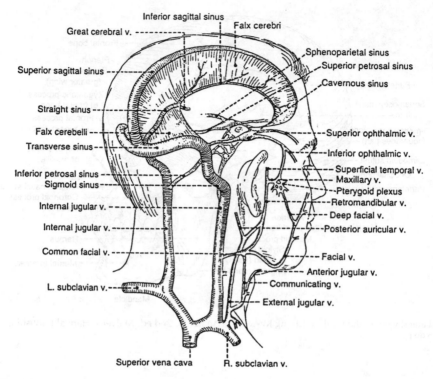

Cranial venous sinuses and veins of the head and neck. In Chung KW. Gross Anatomy, 2nd ed. Malvern, Harwal Publishing, 1991.

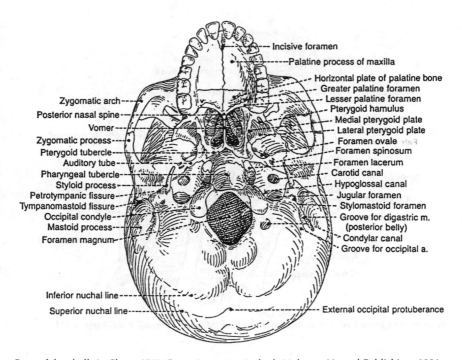

Base of the skull. In Chung KW. Gross Anatomy, 2nd ed. Malvern, Harwal Publishing, 1991.

Appendices

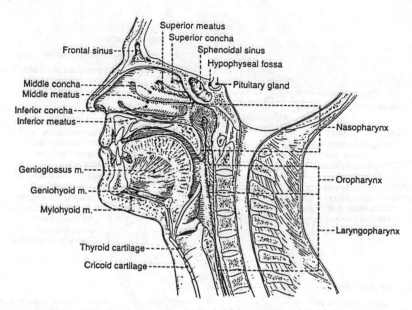

Pharynx. In Chung KW. Gross Anatomy, 2nd ed. Malvern, Harwal Publishing, 1991.

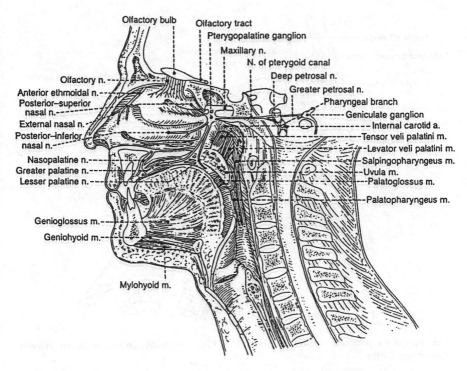

Nasal cavity. In Chung KW. Gross Anatomy, 2nd ed. Malvern, Harwal Publishing, 1991.

Appendices

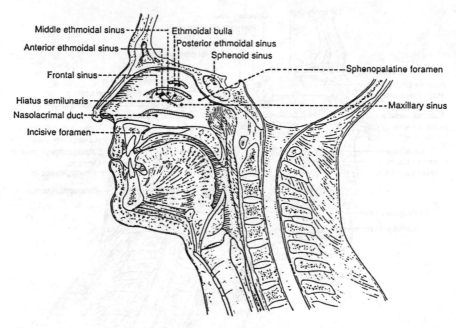

Middle ethmoidal sinus
Anterior ethmoidal sinus
Frontal sinus
Hiatus semilunaris
Nasolacrimal duct
Incisive foramen

Ethmoidal bulla
Posterior ethmoidal sinus
Sphenoid sinus
Sphenopalatine foramen
Maxillary sinus

Openings of the paranasal sinuses. In Chung KW. Gross Anatomy, 2nd ed. Malvern, Harwal Publishing, 1991.

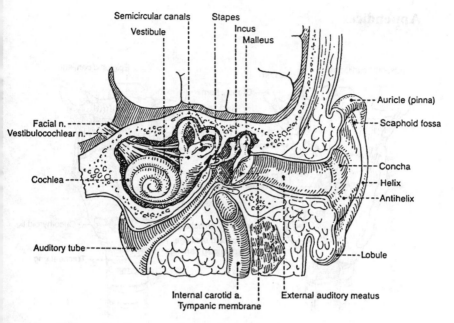

External, middle, and inner ear. In Chung KW. Gross Anatomy, 2nd ed. Malvern, Harwal Publishing, 1991.

Appendices

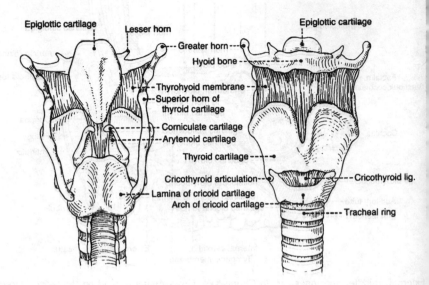

Epiglottic cartilage

Lesser horn

Greater horn

Hyoid bone

Thyrohyoid membrane

Superior horn of thyroid cartilage

Corniculate cartilage

Arytenoid cartilage

Thyroid cartilage

Cricothyroid articulation

Lamina of cricoid cartilage

Arch of cricoid cartilage

Epiglottic cartilage

Cricothyroid lig.

Tracheal ring

Muscles of the larynx. In Chung KW. Gross Anatomy, 2nd ed. Malvern, Harwal Publishing, 1991.